Seven Years Later

SEVEN YEARS LATER

by Catherine Buckler

Copyright © 2024 by Catherine Buckler. All rights reserved.

This book or any portion thereof may not be reproduced or used in any manner whatsoever without the express written permission of the publisher except for the use of brief quotations in a scholarly work or book review. For permissions or further information contact Braughler Books LLC at info@braughlerbooks.com.

The views and opinions expressed in this work are those of the author and do not necessarily reflect the views and opinions of Braughler Books LLC.

Printed in the United States of America

First Printing, 2024

Softcover ISBN: 978-1-955791-90-8

Hardcover ISBN: 978-1-955791-96-0

Library of Congress Control Number: 2023923767

Ordering Information: Special discounts are available on quantity purchases by bookstores, corporations, associations, and others. For details, contact the publisher at sales@braughlerbooks.com or at 937-58-BOOKS.
For questions or comments about this book, please write to info@braughlerbooks.com.

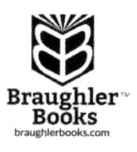

Braughler Books
braughlerbooks.com

This book reflects the author's experiences over time. Some names of hospital personnel and military personnel have been changed.

PROLOGUE

SEVEN YEARS LATER, on March 21, 2012

We are at Moody Air Force Base in Valdosta, Georgia at the Retirement Ceremony honoring Master Sergeant John Buckler. However, John's story really begins in March 2005.

John began his career in the United States Air Force on March 21, 1986. Two years and several duty stations later, he was assigned to RAF (Royal Air Force) Lakenheath England. While in England he married and had two children. In 1990 he was sent to Saudi Arabia for Desert Shield and Desert Storm. After he and his family returned to the United States in 1992, his third child was born.

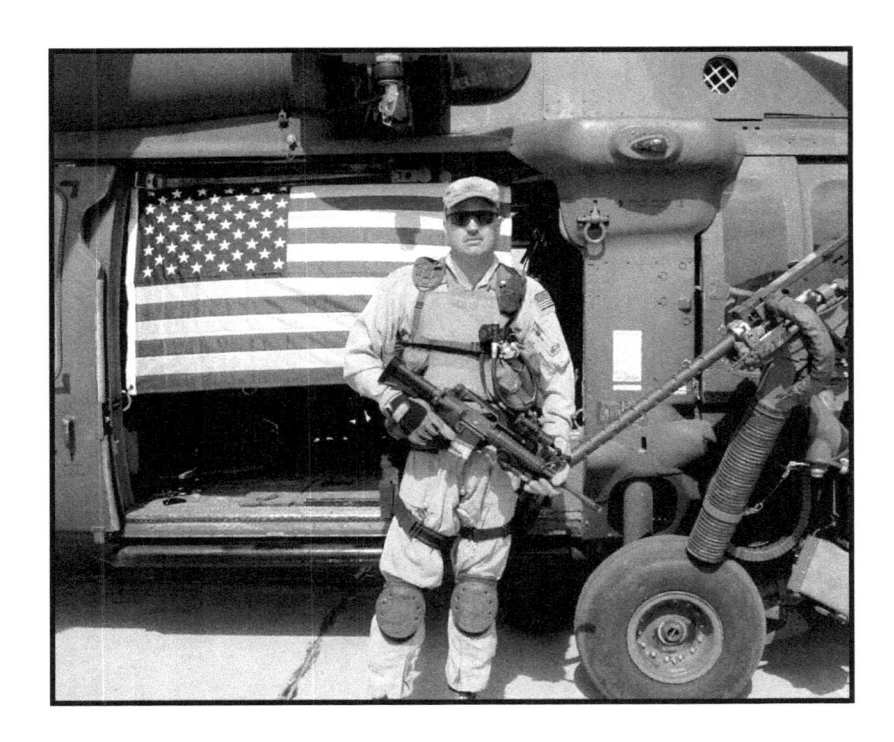

In 1999 he supported Operations Southern Watch, Enduring Freedom and Iraqi Freedom. In 2004 he was assigned to the 56th Rescue Squadron in Keflavik Iceland. During this time, he and his wife divorced.

In 2005 at age 41, he was diagnosed with cancer. He was sent to Lackland Air Force Base in San Antonio, Texas for treatment at Wilford Hall, the hospital on base. I went to be his caregiver. In order to: 1. Keep a record of his treatment; 2. Let everyone back home know what was happening; and 3. Keep my sanity, I began writing emails every week.

The emails proved not only to be helpful to many people (me included) but also provided some life lessons that could be helpful to others going through stressful times.

Some, but not all of the lessons are:

NEVER, NEVER, EVER DENY AN ASPIRATION

BE RELENTLESSLY OPTIMISTIC

IT'S NOT WHAT HAPPENS TO YOU, IT'S WHAT YOU DO ABOUT IT.

NEVER LOSE FAITH

NEVER, EVER GIVE UP

What follows are the emails (some edited for clarification) I sent to friends and family.

Wednesday, April 6, 2005

Dear Family and Friends:

Our son John, who is 41 years old, has been diagnosed with cancer. This is what we know so far.

He is in the Air Force and is currently stationed in Iceland. When he was home on leave for Christmas, he showed us two lumps on his neck and asked what we thought they were. Didn't have a clue but told him he should get them checked out with the doctor as soon as he returned to Iceland.

Don't know how long it took him to go to the doctor but when he finally did was told it looked like overactive lymph glands and to come back if they did not go down. They did not go down and in fact, got larger. The MD did a needle biopsy and said it looked like lymphoma. They then packed him up and shipped him to San Antonio where the Air Force has their equivalent to Walter Reed Hospital, Wilford Hall.

We are told it is the finest the Air Force has to offer and, according to the MDs there, it is the finest in the military. But then everything is relative. It is a teaching hospital so the equipment and knowledge should be state-of-the-art.

They proceeded to take a number of tests including a fine needle biopsy and said it was a cancer but not lymphoma. It is called nasopharyngeal carcinoma of the fossa Rosenmüller. This fossa Rosenmüller is a small indentation above the nose and behind the tonsils. The pharynx is in close proximity. And it has spread to both sides of his neck. It is now a stage III cancer.

On the 13th he will have a port implanted into his jugular and what is termed a "peg" put into his gastro-intestinal tube. The port is to accept the chemo and the peg is for self-feeding. The doctors told him his throat may be too sore for him to swallow or he may be too sick to eat but they do not want him to lose any weight so they will provide him with high-caloric liquids.

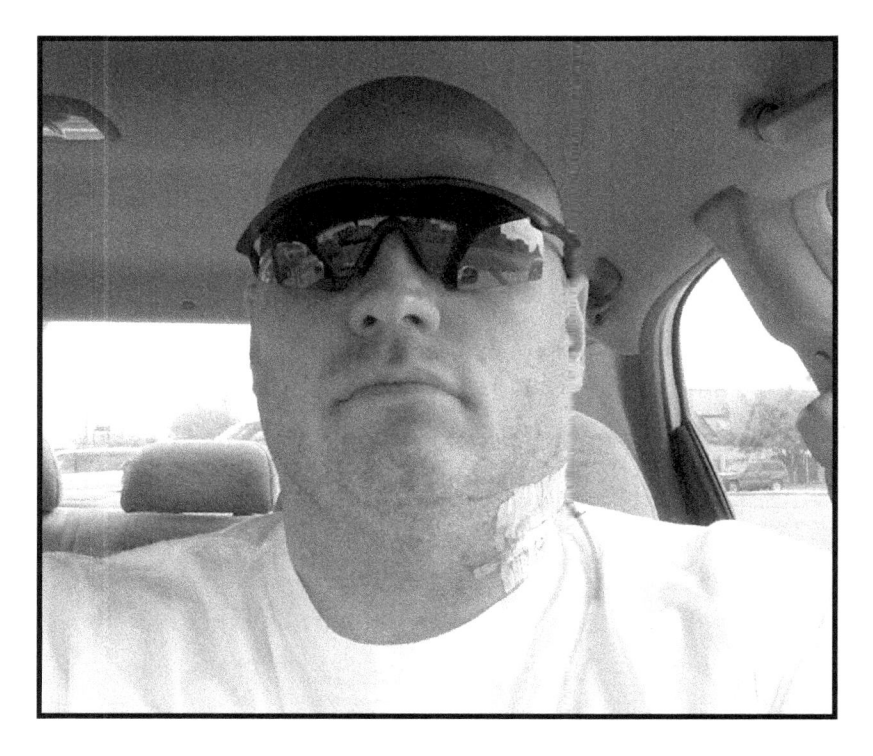

The treatment will be radiation five days per week for seven weeks, concurrent with chemo probably three days per week for one month, then once per week for three months. The prognosis is good in that he has been told that the chances of cure are between 75% and 90%. That is much different from what you read online which is about 35-50%.

This type of cancer is very rare in North Americans. Because their genetic makeup makes them predisposed to getting this cancer, it is common in people of Asian descent. Those North Americans that have gotten it, for the most part, have been exposed to the Epstein Barr Virus which shows itself as Mononucleosis. I seem to recall our three daughters having Mono when they were in their early teens and I think John had it after he went into the service but cannot be sure.

Friday, April 8

Just a bit of the latest news. Ray and I are leaving on Monday afternoon for San Antonio. I will be there indefinitely and Ray must return on the 28th of April as he has some things to take care of and he must be at home to do them.

The most recent update regarding John is that he had an appointment with the dentist and they did a full work-up on him including taking impressions of his teeth, x-rays, and making a shield for him to wear during radiation. He was told the fillings he had in his mouth would burn if they were not shielded from the radiation and therefore his mouth would burn.

There has been a change in the treatment, and I would assume it will change again before it begins. He will begin radiation treatment early next week and every day for seven weeks. Concurrently he will have chemo, I think, three times per week for a month. Then there will be chemo once a week for three months.

Please keep those positive thoughts and prayers going. John's mood is really remarkable. He is confident he is going to get through this as are Ray and I. I was telling someone tonight I am of the opinion that God did not bring John through a major automobile accident when he was a teenager, and a motorcycle accident when he was an airman at Plattsburg, NY, the Gulf War, Afghanistan twice, and

Iraq to take him now. There is something important he must do to have survived all that.

Tuesday, April 12

This morning John went to the dentist and had his teeth examined again, as well as picked up his teeth guards.

John really does not look ill. He does have a good-sized lump on the left side of his neck and a small (quarter-sized) lump on the right side of his neck. He has lost most of his hearing in his left ear. There is an obstruction in the Eustachian tube from the lump. One of the side effects of the radiation is damage to the Eustachian tube. One possibility is he may have permanent hearing loss but also some of the literature suggests this might be a temporary condition.

This afternoon, he went for the radiation simulation. They made a plastic mask of his face, neck and shoulders and marked the sites of the radiation on the mask so they would not have to mark his face. The mask looks like a grate or wide-hole screening. He said he must lie down with the mask on and it is fastened down so he is unable to move. They also put a rope-like something around his wrists which he must hold on to so his arms do not move either.

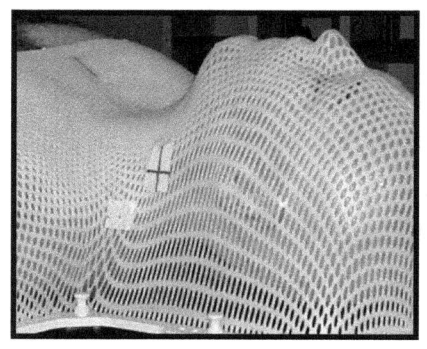

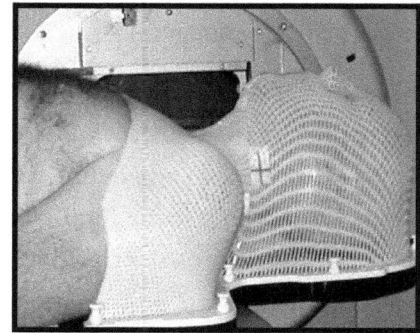

Wednesday, April 13

This morning John went into the hospital to have the port and the peg inserted. He will remain in the hospital overnight then come back to the temporary housing where we are all located. He came through that very well. One of the nurses said he talked all through the surgery. He had to be awake to do whatever the MDs wanted him to do to test the port. About an hour after they were finished, he began to feel nauseous. His neck and stomach were beginning to hurt when he started to get ill. You could just see the color drain from his face. Fortunately, the MD was there and saw this and prescribed some Phenadren. He was taken to his room about 3:30. Once he was settled in, we left as he was really sleepy.

His biggest complaint is that he will not be able to eat until 24 hours past the end of the surgery which means about 2:00 PM on Thursday.

The tumor board met on Tuesday but John was in the simulation when the oncologist called him so he does not know the results of their meeting. He does know that he will have his first chemo treatment on Monday, April 18 at 9:00 am.

His plan right now is to get up and walk for one hour each morning then head to the hospital for his treatment. I hope he can do that as everything one reads suggests that keeping active will help the fatigue that usually hits radiation therapy patients.

Thursday, April 14

John came home from the hospital today, but not until around 3:30. He is feeling kind of puny but doing ok considering everything. He made an appointment with his oncologist for tomorrow morning so we could meet her and ask some questions.

Friday, April 15 - Tax day.

Met with the oncologist and she was able to clarify some things for us. For example, he will have radiation five days per week for seven weeks and chemo one day every three weeks. In other words, he will have chemo on day one, then again on day 22, day 43, etc. This schedule is designed to sensitize John to radiation. There will be a one-month break after the radiation then additional chemo will be done on days 71, 99, and 127. This will be a continuous infusion over four days for three months. Days 71-74, 99-102, and 127-130.

The oncologist looks for John to be here until probably September.

Later today, the radiologist called John and said he would like John to be entered into a "Protocol" or IMRT (intensity-modulated radiation therapy) program. He told John it would be his decision entirely. The advantages to this program are, that it is a different way of doing radiation therapy, more precise/focused. It will require more testing next week. The upside to this is that they are attempting to save his salivary glands. Also, he will have more access to the physicians should he desire. John decided to go for it primarily because the radiologist did not feel there would be a risk in waiting another week to begin the treatment. This, of course, means that the chemo is delayed until the radiation is scheduled. Probably won't begin until the earliest April 25.

Love, Affection and Blessings

K

Monday, April 18, 2005

John met with the radiation department today and was given the following information:

He will be taking part in a Radiation Therapy Oncology Group (RTOG) clinical trial. This research study will use the IMRT planning technique. This study will be monitored by the National Cancer Institute as well as the Institutional Review Board. It is a Phase II study. This treatment plan will try to lower the amount of radiation that the normal tissues receive, while still delivering the desired amount of radiation to the cancer.

There will be an estimated 64 people taking part in this study, with approximately eight people enrolled here at the medical center at Lackland AFB over a period of probably 3½ years.

John will be seen weekly by the Principal Investigator, Dr. Greene, during the radiation therapy treatment, then every three months for the first year, every four months for the second year and every six months for the next three years, then annually for life.

As I said in my earlier email, he will be getting radiation treatment five days per week for six weeks, chemotherapy along with the radiation (Cisplatin) once every three weeks, then 5-FU (5-Fluorouracil) periodically over four-day periods for four to five months.

He will have additional tests done this week, i.e., a chest x-ray, blood tests, another dental exam, MRI, perhaps another CT scan of the tumor, a possible CT scan of the liver if his liver function test is elevated, a bone scan, an EKG, an audiogram and a Sialometry test to measure the amount of saliva he produces.

Naturally, there will be some risks to being in this study. However, the benefits appear to significantly outweigh the risks in that John will be seeing his doctor more often than those not in the study which may lead to the improved ability of early detection should there be a possible progression of the cancer. Should he suffer any of the possible side effects, he will have ready access to possible "anti" drugs.

Ray and I are doing well, as well as can be expected. Ray is about to go out of his mind because there is nothing for him to do in this small apartment. But he does not complain. Of course, my back had to have some attention but other than that, we are ok.

Friday, April 22, 2005

This has been a terribly busy week for John. He has had one test after another. X-rays on Monday, a chipped tooth repaired on Tuesday, a hearing test on Wednesday along with an EKG and a meeting with the dietitian, had the stitches taken out of his "peg" on Thursday, and an MRI on Friday. He was supposed to have another blood test today, but they had to inject him with some type of dye for the MRI so the blood test has been postponed until Monday. On Monday he is also to have a saliva test. There is a particular combination of chemicals that needs to be used for this test and they, here at the hospital, had to send away for the correct ingredients. That is the reason for the delay.

The oncology coordinator, Maggie, (the one who makes all his appointments) still says that the radiation and the chemo will begin no later than Tuesday.

One day this week we all met with Maggie and she was saying how great it was that John is taking part in this study not only for his sake but for the sake of many others who will benefit from John's participation. John's response was "Well, our motto in Search and Rescue is 'These Things We Do So Others May Live.'" I nearly lost it but didn't. That's our John!

So far everyone we have met here on the base has been so very kind and helpful. One of our friends in Cincinnati has a brother and sister-in-law, Arnold and Carole, who live here. Ann arranged for us to get in contact with each other and they have been wonderful. Tuesday evening we all went to the Air Force Band concert which was held because of Fiesta Week here in San Antonio. The concert was wonderful. We all had a great time.

Late this afternoon John's radiation oncologist called to say that John's participation in the Protocol Study has yet to be approved. It seems that all the plans have been submitted but the Principal Investigator, Dr. Greene, has yet to approve it. The oncologist said regardless, John will start the treatment on Tuesday, April 26.

Later we were talking and John said he wanted to ask the doctor what the risk would be if he waited until next week to begin the treatment to see if the approval would come through. If the doctor says it would not be a risk, John wants to wait another week, but that is the absolute limit. According to the MD, in or out of the study, John would receive the same treatment. What we don't know is would he have the same access to the MDs and would he be watched as closely.

He was told on Friday the cause of much of the delay is because he is the first one here on this base to be selected for this study.

Love, Affection and Blessings

K

Sunday, April 24, 2005

We had been looking for a church but the only Evangelical Lutheran Church was more than an hour's drive from here. We left a message for the pastor of that church and he phoned back with a suggestion that we go to a closer Wisconsin Synod Mission. We did and that Mission's Pastor's brother was there. He is also a cancer survivor of ten years and was able to talk with John about his experiences. I think we were just supposed to go to that particular church service so John would meet that young man.

Today Marjorie and her three seed (for those of you unfamiliar with the vernacular, "seed" means children) came to visit. Now understand we are seven people in a one-bedroom apartment. There is one queen-size bed in the bedroom, a queen-size sofa bed in the living room, and a small chair that pulls out into a less than twin-size bed. We decided the four males would sleep in the living room and the females in the bedroom. Poor Taylor (Marjorie's middle child) had to sleep on the cushions on the floor. Oh well, that is family life. It's a good thing we all get along fairly well. They will be here until Wednesday morning, then all of them plus Ray will go back to Cincinnati.

Monday, April 25, 2005

Maggie called this morning to let John know he has an appointment with the radiation oncologist this afternoon at 3:00. That is when we will determine if he is to begin tomorrow or next week.

He still needs another blood test and a saliva test. Ordinarily, the blood test would not be a problem but because they have to take it from the port, there are only a couple of nurses trained to do that and that has to be scheduled when there is time.

We are also waiting for the special compound for the saliva test to arrive. This is a waiting game that could be extremely unnerving but so far John is handling it with ease. He just wants to get started so he can get back to work sooner. John always has been a patient person. Pretty much like his dad.

We had the appointment with the radiation oncologist and he gave us some terrific news. John is definitely in the protocol study. I, for one, am very relieved to know this. It seems the approval for John being in the study was not really approval for John's participation. It was approval for the hospital and doctors to participate. The MD spent nearly an hour with us going over the treatment plan, showing us images of John's skull and the diagrams of where they would be aiming the radiation.

He then went over some of the things we can expect John to experience, such as his mouth and skin being very hot and burning somewhat like a sunburn. We were told he should not put anything on his skin unless he had been given it by the hospital staff. He is to take no over-the-counter stuff for the burn.

He also has a piece of paper he needs to keep with him at all times while under radiation therapy stating he cannot have Pilocarpine nor Amifostine, drugs used generally to protect the salivary glands. If he gets a headache, he can take something like Tylenol but, if it gets really bad, they will prescribe something stronger.

Most of the symptoms should subside within three weeks of the radiation treatment. He may lose his sense of taste but that should return within eight months.

With the Chemo, however, some of the side effects will continue until after the chemo has stopped. Also, the chemo may increase some of these symptoms. There is something called fibrosis which occurs under the skin. It may take many months to resolve.

I asked the doctor if he knew what might have caused this cancer. He said it mostly shows up, as we already knew, in people of Asian descent. And generally, from a virus of some type. Here in the States some of those who have contracted the disease have been heavy smokers and/or drinkers. John is neither of these. The doctor continued that in John's case, it was more than likely a sporadic, random mutation of a cell. In the vast majority of cases, it is due to chance.

John did have the blood test done today, but not from the port as they had wanted to do. It seems the MD took too long to talk with us and the port had not yet been accessed. The saliva test will be done tomorrow morning before they start the chemo. He needs to be at the hospital by 7:45 am.

Maggie tried to call John's cell phone tonight but his phone is not working. She grabbed both of my phone numbers and called our house in Cincinnati to leave a message for John that he is not to have anything to eat or drink including brushing his teeth for one hour before the saliva test. Tracy called me to give me that message and while I was on the phone with her, I get a beep on my cell phone that there was a message waiting. Then a few minutes later Maggie called on the phone that is here in the apartment to give me the same message. The cell phone message was from Maggie also. Is she tenacious or what?

John is so very relieved that this is starting tomorrow. He was getting very antsy but knowing his road to recovery really starts tomorrow he has relaxed somewhat.

The doctor did tell us that this hospital and staff is one of only three here in the whole state of Texas to be approved to do this protocol. He said how many were across the country, but I cannot remember. I do know it is not many.

Now for some really good news or at least I choose to think so. Remember I said John had another MRI last Friday? The doctor received the results of that this afternoon and told us that the folks who read the MRI thought he had already begun treatment because it was different from the first one. The larger tumor was smaller!!!! Not, the doctor said, a lot smaller but smaller. I suggested it was the power of the holy water John's friend Sue had given me for John as well as the power of all the prayers being said for him.

Tuesday, April 26. 2005

We are at the hospital at 7:30. John had the saliva test which he said is a bit more difficult than one might think. He had to hold all the saliva in his mouth for five minutes without talking, moving his tongue, or swallowing. Then spit into a cup, then wait and hold for one minute, spit into the cup again every minute for another five minutes. The doctor then gave him this citric acid solution which he had to hold for 1 minute then spit into a cup each minute for five minutes. When you stop to think about it, it is an automatic action for us to swallow when we have liquid in our mouths.

After this test, he went to the chemo room and they accessed his port and began the chemo. This process took about four to five hours. He finished that about 2:30 then at 3:00 he went to radiology. That process took about an hour due to the fact that they had to get everything set up as it was the first time. He arrived back at the apartment around 4:30. John said he was feeling pretty good.

The doctor had prescribed medication for him to take for nausea so John took what was prescribed. About two hours later he started feeling queasy but took the third pill they also prescribed if the first two didn't work. Well, that didn't work either. He felt bad most of the night.

Bret (Marjorie's oldest) has something called a hacky sack with him. (I thought he said Hackensack and commented it was in New Jersey to which I received "the look"!) The look is like saying "Grandma, you are demented!" But I digress. Bret was out in the courtyard-like area between two apartment buildings (one-level apartments) playing with the hacky sack and kicked it onto the roof. Of course, there is no maintenance person around to get us a ladder, so Bret gets up on a small concrete bench that is outside each apartment, Ray and I help Taylor up on Bret's shoulders, then Taylor pulls himself up so he can barely see over the edge of the roof to find the hacky sack. It was too far for him to reach and besides he is not really comfortable up that high without much support so he gets down while I locate a broom in the apartment. Now we start the process all over again. With success! What we should have done was get John's camera and have a record of this adventure but we didn't. You'll just have to take my word for it, it was quite a sight.

Wednesday, April 27, 2005

We took Marjorie, her three seed and Ray to the airport at 6:45 this morning. John's radiation appointment is at 9:30. From now on he will get this treatment at 10:00 a.m. every day except on the day he has chemo, then it will be in the afternoon. He was finished in 25 minutes today. A nurse in the chemo area gave him some liquids and something to alleviate the nausea and he is feeling pretty good. He had the nurse take his photo with his mask on in several positions so when we get prints made, I'll send them to Ray and you can see them from him.

He is through for the day now and is taking a nap because he did not sleep well last night and had to get up early this morning. I hesitate to say it is because of the treatment he is getting. We'll know more after a few more treatments and after being on a pretty regular schedule.

Love, Affection and Blessings

K

Thursday, April 28, 2005

Last night we decided we would get up early (7:45) and walk for about one hour before John's treatment. He will go in every day at 10:00 am which makes it nice for us to plan the day.

John met with his radiation oncologist and he will meet with him each Thursday.

The only real side effects John has experienced are 1) hiccups and 2) a heartburn-like sensation in his stomach instead of his esophagus. We are not sure what to do about either one. We have tried all the home remedies I know about for the hiccups but nothing works for long. Ice cream works for a while, peanut butter for a while, cold liquids, or a nap for a while, but they come back. We tried an ice-pack on the back of his neck but that was no good either. The MD suggested he try the meds he was to take on an "as-needed" basis for nausea, but that didn't work either. He has to wait until tomorrow to ask if he can take Tums or another antacid for the heartburn-like symptom.

Friday, April 29, 2005

The doctor gave John a new prescription for the hiccups. Who knew there was a script for hiccups? It is called Metoclopramide –

PO. He is to take it three to four times per day 30 minutes before meals. This seemed to work. The hiccups are slowly easing up. It is either the medication or the fact that the chemo is leaving his body. He was also given permission to take Tums if needed.

Monday, May 2, 2005

We had a relatively quiet weekend, or I should say I did. One of John's friends from Moody Air Force Base in Georgia came through here on his way to Albuquerque. He stayed here Friday and Saturday night. On Saturday during the day, he and John went to Fiesta Texas which is an amusement park not unlike Kings Island. I think John really had a good time but probably pushed himself too much as he was really tired both Sunday and Monday.

Tuesday, May 3, 2005

We are into a routine of sorts if you want to call it that. We get up and are out of the apartment usually by 8:15 am. We walk for about 45 minutes. As it turns out we measured it today by car and it is about two and a half miles. John says I am walking too fast for him. Ha! Anyway, we get back home and I fix his breakfast while he changes clothes. After he leaves for the hospital for his radiation treatment (he says there is really no need for me to come along except on the days he sees the doctor,) I do whatever here, dishes, laundry, typing emails or writing cards.

When he gets home, we usually do errands, go to the library to email, go to the post office, commissary (the base grocery store) or whatever. Then it is home and I start dinner. He has really been getting tired so sometimes he takes a nap in the afternoon. We have been eating an early dinner so by 7:30 or 8:00 we are beginning to get hungry again, so it is snack time. This is ok for John as he is supposed to be maintaining or gaining weight. I may have to join a gym when I get home. John has decided he needs to eat less at one time, but more often. I just need to eat less!

Small things are beginning to show up for John because of the treatment. Occasionally he has said he has a metallic taste in his mouth, and the left side of his neck gets stiff. Those things as well as the fatigue all have been expected. He was told his mouth would get sore and he may not be able to swallow because it will hurt. So far none of that has happened. But today was only the sixth treatment. Maybe he will be one of the lucky ones and not have those side effects. The brother of the pastor of the church we are attending said he had none of the usual side effects except for weight loss.

Thursday, May 5, 2005 (Cinco de Mayo)

After the radiation treatment today, John and I met with the doctor. John described one other sensation. The tumor on the right side seems to be more tender and appears to John to be larger. The doctor examined it and suggested he wanted to do another CT scan. He wanted to compare it with the last CT to make sure the radiation treatment plan was targeted in the right place.

We went back to the hospital at 1:00 for the scan. This time he had to wear the mask so he would be in exactly the same position as when he received the treatment. They are really watching him closely. He also had more blood work today. Each week while undergoing radiation, as well as on the day he has chemo, more blood work will be done.

We probably won't know the results of the scan until tomorrow, maybe. The only thing we can assume is if they have to reprogram the treatment plan, we will know tomorrow. We are just praying that the tumor on the right has not gotten any bigger. The one on the left appears to have gotten smaller.

Friday, May 6, 2005

After the radiation today, John told me the following. The tumor on the right side has in fact grown. During the radiation, the technicians put a device, (a diode) over the tumor to measure the amount of radiation that the tumor was receiving. They will know this afternoon if it is receiving the amount called for in the plan. If not, the focus and dosage will have to be increased. He will know for sure on Monday what changes, if any are warranted.

Love, Affection and Blessings

K

Saturday, May 7, 2005

Last evening about 6:00 Dr. Peterson phoned. He is a radiation oncologist. He said the tumor on the right side was getting slightly more radiation than the plan called for and of course, the tumor getting larger was quite rare.

Anyway, the Dr. suggested we wait a short while to see if the tumor does begin to shrink. If in fact it grows, there are a couple of options. One is to give John radiation twice a day which, the Doctor says would be quite hard on John. The other is to call in an ear, nose and throat MD to consider "neck dissection." In plain speak, this is surgery to remove the tumor.

Later last night, John noticed that at the base of his neck at his collarbone, there was some puffiness. We really didn't know what it could be but just something worth noting until Monday when he goes back for radiation.

Sunday, May 8, 2005 (Mother's Day)

This morning John woke up tired, with a headache and a sore throat. This same type of thing happened last Sunday. I don't know if it is because of the radiation or the fact that two of his friends from Iceland stopped in on their way to Albuquerque for training and John went out most of the day Thursday and part of the day on Friday. The weekend before, another friend was here Friday and Saturday.

This morning we went to church and then to the library to do some emailing. We were going out for dinner but I think we are going to forget it for today. There are thunderstorms going on and with John being tired, I would just as soon stay in and wait until he is feeling better. As it turned out we did stay in and ate junk food all day long. Kind of a wonderfully different Mother's Day.

Monday, May 9, 2005

We had a very busy day today between walks, treatment, emailing, post office, etc. We did have an appointment with the chemo doctor, Dr. Gallagher today. She looked at John's blood tests and said everything looked really good. He is having some sinus drainage which she said is because we are in Texas and has really nothing to do with the cancer. That is a surprise coming from sinus valley. She gave John three more medications: one for sinus drainage, Claritin, and two for his sore throat, Sucralfate and something called Triple Mix. It has Lidocaine Viscous, Mylanta II and Benadryl in it.

Of course, he can take none of this without having the radiation oncologist, Dr. Peterson approving it. It seems to us that those two MDs don't speak with one another. Other than that, the doctor says John is really doing well. I am really pleased and only somewhat concerned about the slight increase in the size of the tumor on the right side.

John is also having headaches a couple of times a week. Dr. Gallagher said he could take Tylenol or Midol for that. Something else John has to check with Dr. Peterson about.

John has to be very careful with the sun and it was very sunny and hot today. He has a straw cowboy hat to wear, but he hates it. He came up with the idea to make a ball cap he has with his Rescue emblem on it into a sort of French Foreign Legion hat with a cover that comes down from the hat to his shoulders. He wanted the emblem from his search and rescue squadron on it, green feet, but when we took it to a place here that did that kind of work, they wanted a small fortune just to set up the machine. Then there was a fee for each letter of the title plus who knows what for the feet.

I happen to know someone (some of you know Judi as well) who has a multitude of embroidery machines so I gave her a call. Judi was her wonderful self and said she would be glad to try to do what John wanted. We mailed the material, hat and instructions to her today. What a good friend she is!

Tuesday, May 10, 2005

John checked with Dr. Peterson today and he has been cleared to take the meds prescribed by Dr. Gallagher. Hope this helps his throat and his headaches.

Wednesday, May 11, 2005

Don't know if you heard or would have even paid attention if it was on the news up where you are but there was a helicopter crash in Albuquerque on Wednesday. It carried the pilot, and flight engineer and one more person. The copter crashed killing the flight engineer and injuring the other two. This was to have been the last flight of the pilot and the flight engineer as they were retiring. John knew both the pilot and the flight engineer.

Both of these AF men were instructors at what is called the "Schoolhouse" in Albuquerque. They were flying the same type of helicopter as John flies.

These men are really something. They are a brotherhood unto themselves. When one of them hurts, they all hurt. Still don't know the cause of the crash and may never know for sure.

Thursday, May 12, 2005

John saw the radiation oncologist today and he confirmed what John already knew. The tumor on the right side that he was worried about last week, has in fact shrunk. So, for now, we don't have to worry about having radiation twice a day or surgery. Amen!

He has, however, lost some weight. Neither of us is quite sure how that is possible. He eats, even with a sore throat, just about everything in sight. As an example, yesterday he had a bowl of cereal before we went on our walk. When we returned, he had two scrambled eggs with mushrooms and cheese, some grapefruit and a cup of tea. We went to the library and post office and to the UPS store. While there I said "Let's stop for some ice cream at the BX."

(Base Exchange) Baskins & Robbins. Mmmm! He had a three-scoop chocolate sundae with whipped cream.

When we got home, he was hungry again so had some leftover pork tenderloin and rice. I had made a key lime pie so he had two pieces of that. Later we had dinner, more leftovers, another piece of pie and close to the time to go to bed he had a miniature Dove Bar. Now you tell me how someone who eats like that every day can be losing weight.

We have decided that he should have a Boost Plus, which the hospital provides, each morning before our walk, then eat as he usually does during the day, and another Boost Plus before he goes to bed. He will try that this next week to see if he is still losing.

John has been getting tired more often so every afternoon he tries to take a nap. I cannot remember if I explained the sleeping arrangement before or not, but there is one bedroom and a sofa bed in the living room. Each room has a TV. John absolutely refuses to allow me to sleep on the sofa bed so that is his bed.

However, when he takes a nap, I make him go into the bedroom. Today was a bit different. When we got back this afternoon, he was hungry so had something to eat first. There was a movie I wanted to see with Spencer Tracy and Katharine Hepburn that he is absolutely not interested in, so I said he should let me know when he was ready to lie down and I would come out of the bedroom. That was at about 3:00. I came out of the bedroom about 30 minutes later and there he was, sound asleep on the sofa. Well, I was not about to wake him up so I stayed in the bedroom until I had to come out to start dinner. He slept through my clanging around the kitchen. Finally, he woke up about 6:00! After dinner, I made him promise to sleep in the afternoon in the bedroom. If I have to stay in the bedroom every day, I will go stir crazy!!!

Last week on Thursday two of John's Air Force buddies from Iceland, Chris and Billy, stopped here on their way to Albuquerque. They really are terrific young men. John has said that both have a great sense of humor but that Billy is just a bit demented. Billy is newly married and cannot wait to get to Albuquerque as his bride is also in the Air Force stationed at Nellis AFB in Las Vegas and is going to meet him in Albuquerque. Anyway, John spent Thursday evening with them and on Friday, after his treatment, the four of us went to lunch at Chili's. We had a fun time telling stories on each other but mostly on John.

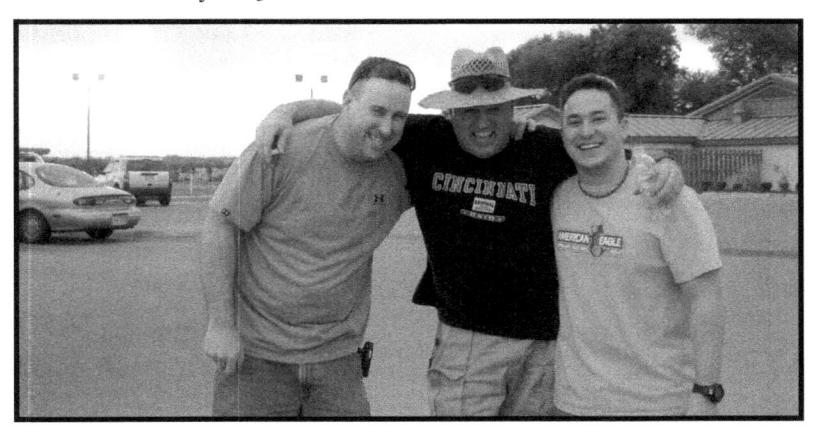

After lunch was over and we are walking to the car, Billy said "John, you have something on the back of your leg." I looked and it was a piece of tomato. I commented that John had not had any tomatoes. How did he get tomato on his shorts when he hadn't eaten any tomato?

After we were in the car Billy said "That reminds me of this guy who got crabs and he didn't even have sex."

Chris: "What are you talking about? What does that have to do with the tomato on John's leg?" John and I are laughing so hard we can hardly see. Billy: "But don't you see, he got it from the toilet!

He didn't have sex!" Chris: "What???? Have you lost your mind?"

K: Laughing so hard I can barely speak, "Billy, unfortunately, I understand what you are trying to say." Thereby confirming what was already suspected. I have now totally lost my mind. Been living in two rooms just a bit too long!

Love, Affection and Blessings

K

Friday, May 13, 2005

This morning I decided we were not going to take a walk as John has a cold. He was running a very slight temperature, coughing and had a runny nose. He slept until after 9:00 AM and we had gone to bed fairly early. He went to his treatment and then we went to the library. Around 2:00 another friend, a pilot on the HH60 helicopters from Iceland, stopped by and they went to lunch. I had already decided not to go. He is probably going to miss his nap today.

John looked on the internet this morning at the library to see if there were any direct flights to Albuquerque next Friday after his treatment. They are going to have a memorial service for the flight engineer who was killed this week. There was no direct flight so it all depends on what time the service is whether or not he will be able to go.

This past week John met another member of this Protocol study. He has cancer somewhere in his neck. Not sure of the exact place. Funny thing is he was a pilot on the F111s that John worked on before he changed rates and became a flight engineer on Search &

Rescue Helicopters. They generally reviewed where they had been and when, and decided they probably were not at the same place at the same time. It is just a bit disconcerting however, knowing they both had something to do with the F111's and both have cancer in the head and neck.

Saturday, May 14, 2005

We did in fact get out today and do some sightseeing. Went to a place downtown called Riverwalk. What a unique place that is. There are restaurants, clubs, bars and shops all along this walk as well as very quiet meditative areas. There are also river boats (pontoon types) that you can take. One takes you on as a shuttle between various places along the river and the other is a narrated ride. We did both. We also walked almost all the way around the river before getting on one of the boats. Most of this river is natural however there is a portion of it that is man-made. This Riverwalk was completed many years ago at a cost of around $440,000.

It is right across the street from the Alamo, which we were going to go to, but it was late, so we decided to come back another time. We were getting a bit hungry and decided to come back close to the base before we ate. Of course, we had stopped to get ice cream so we weren't all that hungry but our feet were beginning to give out.

On the way back south towards the base, we decided we wanted Italian for dinner. Actually, John wanted stuffed shells. We decided we would come back to the apartment and look in the phone book for Italian restaurants, then call to find out if they had stuffed shells. We found one and I called. No stuffed shells, but they did have stuffed manicotti using the same ingredients I put in shells. Where was this restaurant? Back north and past where we had been on the Riverwalk.

This restaurant is in what is called the North Star Mall. It sits in the middle of the shopping mall with the kitchen part on the side where stores would be. Lo and behold, as I look around what do I see? TALBOTS! I love, love, love Talbots. I did not, however, subject John to my desire to run into the store, waving my credit card in my hand. I suggested I would do that another time when he was not with me. The meal was really good. I think we may want to do that again.

Sunday, May 15, 2005

After church this morning we stopped at the store. There was a recipe on the Food Network for a risotto that I thought John would like and be able to eat. Even with the medicine he is getting for the sore throat, it is getting more and more difficult for him to swallow. He loves grapefruit and grapefruit juice as well as orange juice but is no longer able to get it down.

Anyway, this recipe includes rice, mushrooms, onions, garlic and peas. Turns out he really did like it and was able to get it down with relative ease.

We had talked about his keeping up with his physical fitness. He said he wanted to do pushups and had gotten permission from the doctor. He has not done any since we arrived. I thought since he wasn't used to doing them, he should start out slow so I said "OK, get down and give me three!" He just looked at me and laughed. So much for physical fitness.

Monday, May 16, 2005

Today John asked me to make another key lime pie so he could take one into the hospital with him for the chemo nurses. I did and he took it with him when he had his blood work done. He also weighed himself and gained two pounds. That's more like it! Since he was feeling better, I thought about the push-ups again and said "OK, get down and give me five." He laughed out loud and repeated, "Give me five". What's the matter? "Mom, I do 41 push-ups at a time!" That may be nice but I still have not seen one, and from the looks of it, I won't be seeing any, any time soon.

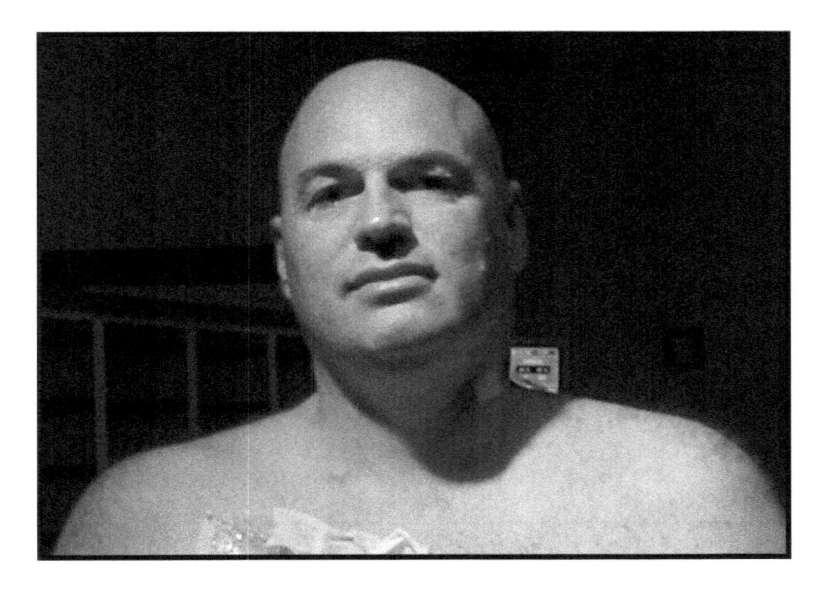

He is having more and more difficulty swallowing and beginning to get sores in his mouth. His sinuses are draining considerably now and he is hacking and coughing a lot. I really think, regardless of what the doctor says, that this is caused by the tumor shrinking and opening up his sinuses so they are able to drain off what has built up over these last few months. I am probably wrong but we will see. He has small marks on his face from the radiation. Also, his neck is getting red as though he has a sunburn and it itches as though from a sunburn. The hospital gave him an aloe gel to use and that is the only thing he is allowed to use. The headaches are not as many any longer, but he still has a cold so he has a cough and a runny nose.

Tomorrow, John will get his second dose of chemo along with the radiation. We anticipate he will get the hiccups again and perhaps feel a bit nauseated but he now has medication for both so perhaps it won't be as bad as the first time.

John has now had 15 radiation treatments. Only 18 more to go.

Tuesday, May 17, 2005

John was gone nearly all day. He had chemo in the morning at 8:00 which lasted for four to five hours, then had radiation. Came home about 3:00. He asked for something he could use for the itch. They will have something for him tomorrow. He is really tired today and his throat is so sore he is unable to eat anything. We had fettuccini Alfredo tonight and he could only take a few bites. He is able to drink Boost but even that is difficult to swallow at times. Tonight, he injected some Boost into the peg for the first time.

Wednesday, May 18, 2005

This morning after our walk, John was hungry so I fixed scrambled eggs. He was only able to eat half, but had a glass of milk to go along with what he did eat. He got the hiccups this morning for about one minute. He decided to try one other home remedy before taking the medicine. He stuck out his tongue and held it between his fingers for about one minute. It seemed to work. At least he did not have them again before he left for his radiation.

If John feels well enough, he is going to play golf with the other person, Mark, who is on the program with him.

John has not been able to eat anything else today. He is trying to drink the Boost but he says everything he puts into his mouth, tastes terrible.

He got the hiccups again this afternoon but this time the new technique did not work. He finally wound up taking one of the pills prescribed for them and so far, so good.

Thursday, May 19, 2005

We saw the doctor this morning and he thinks John is doing very well, even though he lost some weight. If you take into consideration he played golf (nine holes) yesterday, we walked for one solid hour this morning, and he had not had anything to eat, losing a couple of pounds is not too bad.

Dr. Peterson noticed John has a yeast infection in his mouth. This shows up as small sores on the inside of his cheeks and in the back of his throat. He prescribed Fluconazole (Diflucan) to take once per day. This is to alleviate the infection.

Love, Affection and Blessings

K

Thursday, May 19, 2005

Some of you may be interested in what it is like to live on a military or more specifically a United States Air Force Base. You are given a military identification card either for being in the military, being the spouse or dependent of an active-duty military person, or being retired from the military or a spouse of a retired military.

Anytime you are on the base you must have your military ID with you in case you are stopped for any reason. If you leave the base, you must have your ID with you to regain entrance to the base. So far, we have not been stopped.

There is a Commissary where you can buy all your groceries plus non-prescription drugs. There is also a Base Exchange (BX) where they have a mini department store, and a Home and Garden store which sells the usual stuff for the garden, plus furniture and housewares. In the Commissary, BX and Home and Garden store, when you check out you must show your identification as well as in the library before you can sit down to use one of the computers. In the BX there are some mall-like stores, leather, hats, jewelry, as well as some kiosks and a food court. That is sometimes where we go to get Baskins-Robbins Ice Cream.

There is a UPS Store, dry cleaners, movie theater, fitness center, swimming pool, track for walking or running, an 18-hole golf course, a post office and a postal station. The postal station does not mail anything nor sell anything. That is the place we go to pick up our mail. As far as I can determine that is the only reason for their existence. That and the fact that it is on one side of the base and the post office is on the other side of the base.

This is a huge base. To go to the post office, if one doesn't use bridges, one must exit the base, cross a highway and re-enter another gate. The highway is called Military Highway and it runs the full length of the base and then some. There are Interstate Highways all around us so it is fairly easy to get around. The only problem in doing that is similar to Cincinnati in that some streets are named one thing on one side of the street and something else on the other. At one intersection, a normal four-street intersection, the streets have three different names.

There are some fast-food places on the base, (Burger King, Popeye Chicken, Godfather's Pizza,) one restaurant, a bar-b-que place that is only open for lunch, a Bank of America and a credit union. There is the officer's club and the enlisted club as well as a place called Fisher House which is similar to the Ronald McDonald House. And of course, the hospital, Wilford Hall. There is also a legal office, a dental office, a medical multimedia building, etc., etc., etc. Not to mention all the living quarters for all those permanently assigned here, and the flight line, runways and hangars for all the aircraft, Parade grounds, and a hotel for guests of those recruits who are graduating. There is a graduation every Friday with a parade and a band. The whole nine yards. This is a city within a city surrounded by barbed wire fence.

It took a while for me to find my way around the base but I am fairly adjusted to it now. I have to have John go with me the first time I go somewhere off base so I will feel comfortable going by myself. Should John get permanently assigned here and not have his trailer, we would be living in another different area called base housing. That would not be bad but if we get assigned to one of those places, John would have to mow the lawn at least once a week. The lawn is not allowed to get any longer than two inches. With all the rain they have here, that could be a problem.

Then there is reveille, retreat and taps. Reveille happens at 6:00 am, retreat at 5:00 pm and taps at 9:00 pm. If you are outside at any of these times, walking or driving, you must stop until the music stops including the National Anthem. If you are walking you must either face the nearest flag or the area from which the music is playing.

Then there is the loudspeaker system. Not only do they play reveille, retreat and taps, but when there is a thunderstorm within five miles of the base, they announce that as well. Then when the storm has passed, they announce an all-clear. That is very good if you need to prepare for the storm, BUT, they announce this at all times of the day and night. We have been awakened at 4:00 am to hear the all-clear. This is not music; it is a voice speaking through the loudspeakers. Just what I want to hear at 4:00 am, "The storm has passed...." Thank you for that!!

This week the Commissary is having a "case sale" where if you buy a case of something you get a special price. You know if I was at home, I would be stocking up but there is just no place here to store anything. The prices are pretty good at the Commissary on most items. At least they are cheaper than at home and on the base, you do not pay any sales tax even for non-consumable items. I can't compare prices here in San Antonio because I have only been to one of the area supermarkets once or twice and that was for key lime juice which they don't carry on base. When checking out at the Commissary there are people who bag your groceries and then take them to your car for you. They work only for tips so there is quite a rivalry for those packing jobs.

There is a store called Class 6. I don't understand the name because it is a liquor store.

I mentioned before the name of this hospital is Wilford Hall. Called affectionately by Air Force personnel as Big Willy. This place has, I think John said, 16 miles of hallways. There is almost anything you need to survive in the basement which is where John gets his radiation and chemo treatments. There are several offices in this area as well as a conference room plus the treatment rooms. In addition to the treatment rooms, there is a huge waiting room complete with bathroom facilities and TV. There is another waiting room for the radiation treatment folks and in there we have a TV whose channels one can change to their liking. With cable of course. Also, the chairs are very comfortable. Down the hall is the chapel and beyond that on another hallway is a dry cleaner, a post office, the dietitian/nutrition area, a Shopette which has all kinds of food items, magazines, baby items, hygiene items, etc. Beyond that is a snack shop, a coffee shop and a full cafeteria. I went to the cafeteria today for the first time as we were there in Big Willy from 8:00 AM until after 1:00 PM. I just had a salad and water and the total was 87 cents. Works for me. Good but does not compare to the grilled veggie salad at the Works. (For those not in Cincinnati that is a terrific restaurant run by a local young man in Loveland and their food is terrific.) Can't wait to get there again. Are you listening Joan B? In another hallway is a huge auditorium. Another hallway leads to a full-size pharmacy with a huge waiting room across the hall, TV included, plus other medical facilities. I have not explored the entire basement area but I know there are other nooks and crannies that hold a multitude of different functions.

Friday, May 20, 2005

Last night John wanted to get out of the apartment and off the base so we decided to go to the Tower of the Americas. It looks similar to the space needle in Seattle or the one in Las Vegas. The grounds around it are beautiful, park-like settings, waterfalls, benches and many trees. It is located downtown. We went up to the observation deck and that was quite a sight. It looked as though if it had been a really clear day we could have seen to Houston. We walked around the deck twice, once inside and once out.

When we returned to the apartment, John was hungry as was I so he asked me to make mashed potatoes. He had a box of POTATO FLAKES he wanted me to use. Can you believe it? Well, I knew I was challenging my culinary skills to do this but I gave it the old college try. I added some cheese, Italian seasoning and butter. He ate two servings by himself. I guess I met the challenge.

Today John was feeling pretty well except for those darned hiccups. They go away for a while then return with a vengeance. Even the medication the doctor gave him isn't working. John thinks it might be the nausea medication that is keeping them around. He is drinking a lot of liquid trying to flush the chemo out of his system.

We stopped at the post office this afternoon as usual and you won't believe what was waiting for us. Six pints of Graeter's Ice Cream! I'm telling you I really am going to be thunder-thighs by the time I get home if this keeps up.

Late this afternoon we decided John was feeling well enough to get away for the weekend. We went to Fredericksburg which is about two hours north of San Antonio. It was initially settled by Germans and the German influence is very much a part of the culture as well as the architecture and the shops. When we tried to get a room at the hotel however, it was impossible. Every room was booked. We decided to go about 20 miles away to a place called Kerrville. Found a room there. Fredericksburg is quite a tourist attraction, particularly on the weekends. We plan on returning there tomorrow.

We went to dinner at a place called the "Jefferson Street Café." They were so very accommodating. They cooked a chicken breast for John then put it in the blender. The waitress was very friendly and was telling us that Kerrville has more retired millionaires than Sun City. Also, a lot of snowbirds which should not but does surprise me. The area is in what is called "Hill Country" and it really is pretty. Probably the prettiest part of Texas. We were looking at a book they had there about ranches for sale and they were very expensive. Sort of in the gazillions. When we left the restaurant, we looked back at the entrance and the sign that had said OPEN when we arrived now said SHUT. Cracked me up.

Sunday, May 22, 2005

Yesterday we walked around Kerrville a bit then drove over to Fredericksburg. There was an antique car show going on that John wanted to see so we stopped there first. We should have known better, at least I should have known better. It was 97 degrees but there was a breeze. Anyway, the heat got to John and we left after about an hour. He did have his hat on and a bottle of water but that really didn't help as it was so hot and humid.

We stopped and had something to eat at a German restaurant and bakery where he ate pretty well, then headed home. John rested for about two hours then decided he was hungry so we went to eat again. Does it seem to you our life revolves around eating? We don't eat to live; we live to eat!

Monday, May 23, 2005

John woke up this morning very lethargic. He was up several times hacking and coughing up the mucus and drainage from his sinuses. He says it feels as though he has hit a brick wall. He was very weak. He did eat and drink something but felt as though he had both constipation and diarrhea. Can't quite figure out how that works! He was feeling weak in the knees and lightheaded. I wound up driving him to his treatment this morning and as soon as we got home, he went to bed.

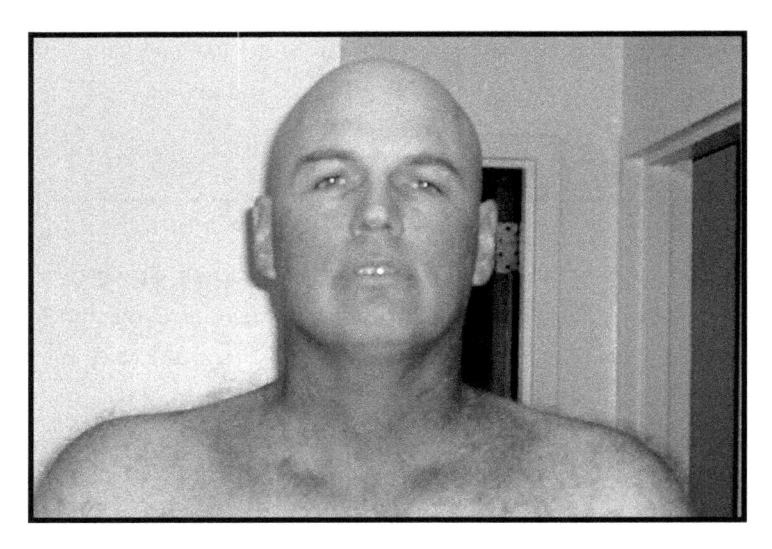

His face, below the eyes and neck, is very red. It looks as though he has a sunburn but he does not. He now has two different medications to use. One is called Biafine. It is a radiodermatitis emulsion. The other is Hydrocortisone Cream 1%. It is an antipruritic anti-itch compound. He is to use these three times per day alternating with each other. His skin is beginning to flake and he is starting to lose his beard. (Falling out.) He says his body is experiencing a whole new set of sensations.

Obviously, we did not walk this morning and I am afraid it will be too hot this afternoon to walk. Perhaps if he feels better this evening we can walk for a bit.

At the hospital this morning, we saw Janie, the wife of Mark, the other person in the program. She said Mark had a bad weekend also and he is a week behind John in the treatments. Perhaps it is the weather because it has been so very hot. We were told this is normal for this time of the year. If that is right, I cannot wait for July and August.

John slept until just before time to keep an appointment this afternoon with the chemo oncologist, Dr. Gallagher. Before each appointment, his blood pressure is taken as well as his weight and temperature. He has dropped six pounds since Thursday!! Even eating!!

We do know he was dehydrated on Saturday and the diarrhea is probably the cause. The doctor was not really concerned with the weight loss but did not like it too much. She is assuming the dehydration is the primary cause. Told him to rest and do nothing, not even walking for a couple of days. We came home and he had half a bowl of soup and something to drink and went back to bed.

Tuesday, May 24, 2005

John slept last night until around 6:00 pm. When he woke, he did not feel much better. He tried to eat but couldn't and only drank a small amount. He did inject himself with some Boost, but again not much.

This morning he at first, was going to walk to his treatment but then decided I should drive him. We ran into Maggie at the hospital and told her how he was feeling and she arranged for him to get some fluids through his port. The nurse in that area decided it would be a good idea for him to have a blood test. A good thing she did as almost all his readings were in the toilet, so to speak. He could have been in renal failure had he not had the blood test, so says the nurse. No wonder he was feeling so punk. He received two bags of fluids. After the first bag they had to stop because he had an appointment with the ophthalmologist. We went upstairs for that appointment and they dilated his eyes. He waited for an hour and the doctor still had not seen him. Evidently, the doctor had some type of emergency. In the meantime, the nurse from the chemo lab downstairs in the basement (where he gets his fluids) called and said he had to get back downstairs for his second bag of fluids. After getting back downstairs and talking with the nurse, John decided she could cancel his appointment with the ophthalmologist. We did not get back to the apartment until 3:45 pm.

He immediately went to bed. I had some errands to do so I left him for about one hour. He got up about 7:00 pm. This time he seemed to be hungry so he ate a small amount, which is what he is supposed to be doing anyway. He also had three glasses of fluids.

I had been invited to play bridge the next day by my friend's sister-in-law, Carole. I told John I was not going to play if he didn't feel any better. He, I think, is trying to get as much into his system so he will feel better tomorrow so I will feel more comfortable leaving him for a few hours. Who is the parent here????? We are still arguing about who is sleeping where. He still refuses to let me sleep on the sofa bed. His argument is "I sleep in it (the bed in the bedroom) during the day and you sleep in it at night."

Even though he is our youngest, and says he is back to being five years old again, he refuses to listen to his mother. And he towers over me so I don't feel as though I am in control. When do they ever learn that usually, mother knows what is right for them!

Wednesday, May 25, 2005

John was up and feeling much better today so I decided it would be ok for me to leave him to play bridge. Had a really good time. There were four tables set up in (are you ready?) the Jack-In-The-Box hamburger place. Evidently, this group plays there every Wednesday. Met some very nice people and played relatively ok considering it has been a while. Was even invited to play again right here on the base at the officer's club next month. If John is ok, I might just do that.

When I got home, John was asleep. He got up around 5:00. Said he received two more bags of fluids. He ate a slightly larger dinner tonight and is really concentrating on taking in more fluids.

Thursday, May 26, 2005

This morning we went to the hospital for his treatment only to find out the radiation machine was not working. This is a brand-new machine and is still getting the kinks worked out of it. Anyway, it is also the day John is to meet with Dr. Peterson, so they said he should meet with the MD while waiting for the machine to get back up. We saw the doctor and he seemed pleased with the way John has come back since Tuesday. John has also gained two pounds since Monday. That's pretty good news.

One of the nurses got the other doctor, Dr. Gallagher, to write John a prescription for Gelclair. This is a compound that he is supposed to swish in his mouth and gargle but not swallow about one hour before eating. This is to help him to swallow without any pain and it is supposed to last for seven hours or more. The Triple Mix that he is currently using makes his mouth numb so this might be better.

As both of these are new medications, he needed to get approval from Dr. Peterson. The doctor approved. Next on the list of things to do today was get more fluids injected. Since the machine still was not back up around noon, he went to have fluids put in and I said I would go to the library. I came home and had lunch, cleaned up the refrigerator and left about 2:00 pm. It had turned so hot and humid that I turned the car around and went to the hospital because it was entirely too hot for John to be walking home.

When I got there, he was getting his radiation treatment. He still had another bag of fluids to get but I just stayed. The nurse said the recent (today's) blood test showed a marked improvement over Tuesday. The only thing that was down was the potassium level. When they gave him the fluids, they gave him a bag with extra potassium. When we left around 3:30 it had stormed and really cooled off a lot. We decided to go right to the library. When we got there the computers were turned off because of the bad weather. We left and went to the post office.

There were two packages for us. One was John's hat. He loves it. It is exactly what he wanted.

The other package is from a delightful person whom I don't want to embarrass by naming but she is terrific. She sent Skyline Chili, Montgomery Barbeque Sauce, LaRosa's Sauce, two magazines and two books.

This has surely been a kind of emotional roller-coaster ride for John and me this week. I sure hope we don't go through something like this again very soon. He is going to get more fluids again tomorrow to hold him for over the long weekend. This weekend we are staying pretty close to here. Way too much traffic on this holiday weekend for us to be out and about.

Love, Affection and Blessings

K

Sunday, May 29, 2005

This has been a relatively quiet weekend. On Friday John had two additional bags of fluids injected into him. We really didn't do much because he was trying to rest to build up his strength. His throat is good some days and not so good others. As an example, Saturday we went shopping at the mall I mentioned earlier, you know, the one that has Talbots. Yes, I did some shopping. Anyway, he had said he was going to take me out to dinner and the Cheesecake Factory is in this mall so that is where we went.

He ordered Shepherd's Pie. He thought it was going to be fixed as they do in England and of course, it was not. It was good but had chunks of meat instead of a small grind of ground beef. He ate some, but not all. Of course, who can finish anything from the Cheesecake Factory?

This morning his throat was so sore as well as his mouth, he could not get anything down except his medications for the soreness. Yesterday, he was ok and today he can't eat. The other person, Mark had a terrific day yesterday, was able to eat everything with no trouble. Today all he has done is gotten sick. He is not able to keep anything down.

After church John said we should try to put some of his leftovers into the blender. We did and he was able to eat a small portion. Incidentally, it looked so gross, I could not watch him eat it. But then I guess you can get used to anything.

Tuesday, May 31, 2005

What a lazy day we had yesterday. We did not put our heads out the door. Stayed in and vegged out on the sofa watching the tube, mostly war movies, played cribbage (for the first time I beat John three games to none) ate some, John mostly drank Boost and other liquids. His throat was a bit more sore but he was able to eat some.

John is now off to get his treatment. Again, this morning, his throat is very sore. He has started taking a Percocet in the evening and again in the morning. This really helps him to eat at least a little. It also helps with his neck. The collar of his shirt rubs against his neck and that is where he is very tender because of the radiation.

The new medication mentioned last time, Gelclair, does not seem to be doing what it is supposed to do as far as helping the sores on the inside of his mouth. But he is going to give it some time.

I have been cooking things I have never cooked before thinking he might be able to eat them. A lemon curd pudding and sweet rice pudding, as examples. He is able to eat those things, however, he can't taste very much right now. I really think this is therapeutic for me. It sort of takes my mind off things, and also gives me something to do in this small apartment.

Wednesday, June 1, 2009

Last week we received yet another package from a friend who had been in China. She sent an incense burner and incense that she bought at a temple in China. While she was there, she was able to speak to the monks and told them about John. They immediately put his name on a tablet for prayers to be said for him and they said a prayer for him right then. Later John said to me, something about why did I think all these people were praying for him, in China, in England, in the Vatican and here in the states. He was also wondering why, when he was no one special was he getting cards and get well wishes from people he didn't know. I said it was because he was cute. He just gave me one of "those looks."

Thursday, June 2, 2005

Today we went for his treatment and we were supposed to meet with the doctor, however, he had had an emergency so one of the nurses asked us if we could come back around 1:00 for the meeting. We came home and had lunch then returned to the hospital. Dr. Peterson did a bore-scope type of thing in John's nose. First, he sprayed a nasty tasting liquid into John's nose, then inserted a long tube with a light on the end into his nose. I really don't know what he was looking for but he commented on how red and raw John's throat looked. John has indicated, when asked by the nurse and the doctor both, without the Percocet his pain level on a scale of one to ten is probably a four and with the Percocet about a one or two.

Dr. Peterson asked if he would rather take a liquid medication (drug) instead of a pill and of course, John said yes. He gave him a prescription for liquid morphine. The doctor said this medication has no Tylenol in it, it is just the straight drug. After we got home, John went straight to bed while I went to the post office, the library and the store.

During our first trip to the hospital this morning, the nurse asked how bad the pain was on his neck. That too is very sore. He is starting to peel and it is getting very difficult for him to turn his head in either direction. They said his skin will begin to weep and when it does, he should put on yet another combination of stuff. The first is Biafine, which he already uses on his neck, then cover that with something called Kaltostat Fortex. It is a Calcium-sodium alginate wound dressing. That is a gel-type compound that will ease the soreness. Then he is to cover that with something called ClearSite. It too is a wound dressing. In addition, they also gave him a cloth-type thing to put around his neck when he begins to use these latest products.

We also saw Maggie today and she said John's blood test taken Tuesday looked very good. All the counts were within the normal range except one that, under ordinary circumstances would indicate an infection. However, she says that it usually shows up that way in cancer patients receiving radiation and chemotherapy. She was not at all concerned. She was concerned, however, about John traveling so soon after the end of his radiation treatment which is on June 10th. We had decided to return to Cincinnati when there was a break in his treatment.

She thought John was going to drive to Valdosta when we left here on the 14th and when we corrected that she was very much relieved. We have changed our plans but I think it just makes sense. The current plan is for Marjorie to fly down to Valdosta and pick up John's two boys and bring them back to Cincinnati. His daughter, Gemma, is in England and won't be back until sometime in early July. Instead of us flying to Atlanta and having to make sure John and his boys can get on the same flight to Cincinnati, we will fly directly to Cincinnati and his seed will already be there. He will then be rested enough by the 25th to begin his drive to Valdosta with Ray to pick up his trailer and drive to San Antonio. Don't know how long Ray will be staying in the trailer after I get here. I kind of think it won't be too long.

We have to be back here on the 1st of July for some blood work he will need done in addition to blood work done while in Cincinnati. He will have to go to Wright Patterson Air Force Base in Dayton to have that done. Maggie is also going to try to make arrangements for him to get some fluids while he is at Wright Pat.

When we do get back here, we will be living in his 32-foot trailer. I don't know how I am going to adjust to that. I have never lived in a trailer and never really wanted to. I know it will be much smaller than this apartment and I am sure I will have some terrific stories to tell in my emails about this new and wonderful adventure.

John is up now and says he is feeling as though he is getting another cold. I checked and it was on May 12 or 13th when he started a cold. At that time, it was about three weeks after his last chemo treatment and this time it is the same time since his last chemo treatment. Hmmm, wonder if there is a connection.

We don't have any particular plans for the weekend. John would like to see Star Wars. Just my cup of tea. I think we are going to try to get Mark and John to go together while Janie and I shop. It's a thought but we'll just have to play that by ear.

Love, Affection and Blessings

K

Sunday, June 5, 2005

On Friday John went to his treatment alone and then received fluids. He was supposed to go to the patient squadron to try to get someone there in contact with Dr. Gallagher. It has something to do with getting him stationed here permanently. (Called PCS'd.) Unfortunately, the office was closed because of a retirement ceremony so that will have to wait until Monday.

His neck now looks like raw meat; it is so very red. The skin is also very tight and he cannot move his head from side to side. He has to move his whole body to look sideways. But it still is not weeping. And the sores in his mouth are still there. I do have to say, however, he has not complained once. Only says things like, "I can't eat any more of that." or, "The shirt collar is really bothering my neck."

The good news is he has had 28 treatments so far and only five left to do, God willing. After that the healing process should start immediately on his neck, throat and mouth. I can't wait until he can eat regular food again without pain. And I am sure he feels the same if not more so.

Saturday we had a terrific day. Mark and John decided to go see Star Wars. It was playing at a theater in what is called the Quarry. Janie and I shopped while the guys were at the movies. We really had a good time. After the movie was over, we ate at J. Alexanders. John was able to eat a cream soup and mashed potatoes. Mark was able to get down some salmon. It is really strange that Mark can drink very cold stuff but John has to have it room temperature; Mark can eat hot food but John's must be room temperature.

When we got home John and I played some Cribbage again (I lost) but he got really tired so we went to bed. I couldn't sleep so I watched TV again until about 2:00 am. I heard John hacking and coughing most of the night.

This morning he was still so tired, he just did not feel up to going to church. I went while he took a nap. They had a birthday cake there for the pastor's daughter, another member of the church, and John. I brought home a piece for him but I am not sure he will be able to eat it. (John's birthday is June 6th, tomorrow.) They all said they were praying for him and for a speedy recovery as I know all of you are as well. We had been invited to the pastor's home to have a cookout for their daughter's birthday, but I had to decline.

Monday, June 6, 2005

Today is John's birthday but it did not start out to be a very good one. He has started to take one Percocet at bedtime but it wears off before 5:00 AM. Consequently, he is up hacking and coughing from that time on. Today his mouth is very sore around his back molars, so sore that he can barely open his mouth.

It started a bit strange for me as well. Most of you know I wear contact lenses. Well, this morning I put both lenses in the same eye. I thought I never would get them separated.

When we got to the hospital this morning, there was a sign posted that Dr. Peterson wanted to see all his patients today. After the radiation, we met with the doctor and he even had a hard time looking into John's mouth. When the doctor first walked into the room, John said "Uncle." The doctor knew immediately what was going on. He has prescribed a patch that John can wear that will last for two to three days with a pain killer in it. Morphine, I think. Anyway, he can use that as well as take Percocet. We are hoping that will help. Can you imagine what all of this would be costing if John were not in the military? I don't know how people do it that do not have excellent health insurance.

While we were with the doctor, he tried to discourage John from leaving town so soon. He wants him to wait a full week or two. John is about jumping out of his skin to get to Cincinnati because his children will be there and he has not seen them for six months. He is not about to wait another week. We explained that he would be near Wright Patterson AFB and our whole family would be there to be caretakers so the doctor said something to the effect "OK, if you feel you will be ok." Then gave us the name of the doctor he should see at WP AFB.

The nurse that got John the Gelclair asked if it was working and when we said it wasn't she recommended he wait to use it until the treatments are over. It may do more good then than now because the mucositis gets more aggravated each time he gets a treatment.

John said today that I would be cooking for myself for the rest of this week and into next as he does not think he will be able to get anything down his throat, not even soup until after the treatments have ended. He will be using the peg from now on, or as he and Mark now say, "Feeding Junior." And I will get an opportunity to lose some weight maybe!!!!!

Tomorrow John gets chemo again so today they are doing an EKG as well as giving him more fluids. He has lost three pounds and is now down to 197. (Of course, the other scale weighed him at 198.) I still don't think that is too bad considering what he has been through. While he was finishing up with the fluids all the nurses in the oncology/hematology lab that were available, came in, stood around John and sang Happy Birthday to him. He really got embarrassed. I did have to laugh as one of the nurses when they finished, said "Aren't we pathetic?" I had to agree. But it was the thought that counted. They all signed a card for him as well.

Tuesday, June 7, 2005

Today when John was weighed in, the scale registered 200. Go figure. Before John's chemo treatment, the nurses drew blood and discovered his counts were all low. Of special concern was the white cell count. Not low enough to stop the chemo treatment but low enough that they are going to give him Neulasta tomorrow. This drug stimulates your body to produce more white blood cells. He will only need one injection of this drug. It is not something he has to take on a regular basis. The nurse mentioned his ANC being down. I don't know if that is the same as the white cell count or not. Those of you who are in the medical field will know. All I do know is they are watching very closely and when something is less than normal, they are on top of it immediately.

Maggie also stopped to talk with me and told me that Dr. Peterson still is very concerned about John going home next week. Once I told her John's sister is an RN and we were within 45 minutes of WP AFB, she said OK but with lots of reservations and warned me that he may not begin to feel better until two to three weeks after the last radiation treatment. I just hope he understands that and realizes he may not be able to do what he is expecting to do with his boys.

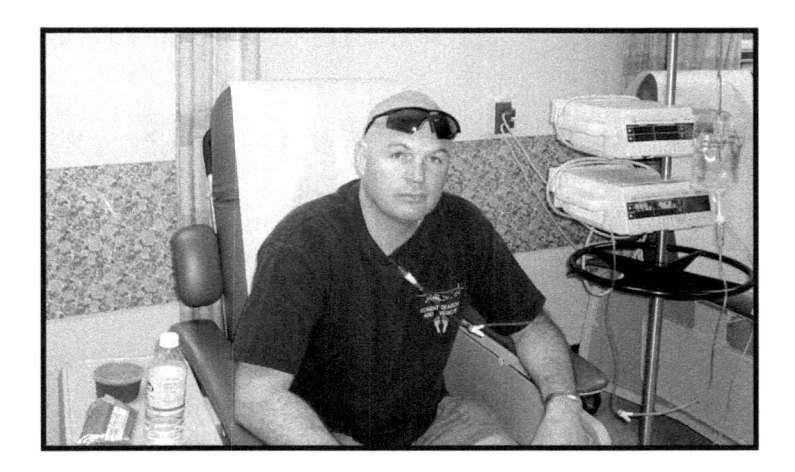

After his radiation and chemo today, John seemed to be feeling better. Not ready to leap tall buildings but better. At least he did not come back to the apartment and crash. He wanted to go to the library which we did. He had some Boost first. This was his third can today. When we came back, he had another can. Hopefully, he will have at least six today.

Wednesday, June 8, 2005

This morning after John woke and sort of dressed, I walked into the living room to find him sitting on the sofa posed somewhat like "The Thinker." Asked, "What are you doing?" Answered. "Thinking." "About what?"

Got sort of the following answer: "About the truck and what I have to do to it when we get back. About the last three treatments. Abraham Lincoln."

"Abraham Lincoln?" Has he had too much Percocet or what? "Yes, I was staring at the carpet and suddenly the face of Abraham Lincoln appeared on the carpet. Then I blinked my eyes and his face disappeared and Julius Caesar appeared facing the other way."

OK, then. Just another day in the life……Went on to the hospital for the 31st treatment. I had an appointment to get my hair done so after his radiation I left while he got his fluids and the shot of Neulasta. I knew he would be at least two hours so I felt comfortable leaving.

Tonight, John also started with the hiccups again. He has not tried the medication yet but maybe he will now. I started to ask him a question about what, I forget, and he told me I was pinging. Pinging? What the heck is pinging? In his dictionary it means worry. So ya think we have had just about too much togetherness or bonding? Can't wait for July, August, and September! I may just stay in Loveland and let Ray deal with it for a while. I'd like to know if Ray starts "pinging."

Later tonight John fed Junior a can of Boost. About half an hour later, he decided he wanted to keep ahead of the fluids so he fed himself some grapefruit juice. I did not think grapefruit juice was a good idea but dreaded the thought of being told I was "pinging" again, so as any good mother would do, I kept my mouth shut. Guess what? Not more than 10 minutes passed when he lost it all. He thinks he won't be doing that again anytime soon.

Thursday, June 09, 2005

Today did not start out too well. First, he woke up about 3:30 am and needed some pain medication. I heard him get up so I did as well. He went back to sleep and I didn't. Turned on the tube and started flipping. Outside of TCM which had an old Barbara Stanwyck movie, every channel had an infomercial. I went back to the movie and finally went back to sleep around 5:30.

When John got up at about 8:00, he was feeling pretty punk. Again, after he had some Boost, he lost it. We went on to the hospital and they gave him some fluids immediately as well as some anti-nausea medicine. After his treatment and after the fluids finished running, we started back to the apartment. On the way, he was sick again. So much for the anti-nausea medication.

He is still constipated so I had to run to the store to get some magnesium citrate to use along with the Senecot. Hopefully, that will help. Of course, he has had no solid food since Sunday when he ate part of the leftover mashed potato he brought home from J. Alexander's. With him losing his cookies now I am sort of glad he has no solid food in him. If no one else knows this, my family knows I am totally unable to cope with someone throwing up. If I don't look at it, I can be ok. So that is what I do. Some caregiver, huh? He is now taking a nap while I do laundry again. Trying to keep up with it before we go home.

His supervisor, Captain Lawrence, phoned today to let him know he would be passing through Lackland tonight. He is going to call if he gets in early enough and they can have a talk. John is just not up to going out and since he cannot eat anything anyway there is no point. He is also too weak to be going to Fiesta Texas. I saw Janie earlier and we may be going to get some Chinese tonight since Mark is also on a liquid diet through the tube.

Tomorrow is his LAST radiation treatment. Hip, Hip, Hooray. I know he will be glad that this part of the treatment is over. Of course, everyone at the hospital is saying he is going to get sicker next week because the radiation will still be working. Let's pray he is going to be unique and will at least be ok on Tuesday. If he can have all this other rare stuff why not that as well?

He found out today that he will be transferred here permanently effective July 1st. Permanent only until the treatment is over and he is given clearance to return to Moody Air Force Base, in Georgia. I think he is not too pleased partly because he will be losing quite a bit of pay. I didn't realize how much is involved in this type of transfer. Under ordinary circumstances, all of his belongings would be shipped here from Iceland. And he would have packed them up himself. However, there is no room here for all of his stuff, so he has to make arrangements for someone in Iceland to pack up his belongings and ship them to Moody. Then he has to make arrangements with someone in Moody to make sure they get stored there until he returns which probably won't be until late October or November. Doing this long distance and not being on-site himself can cause "pinging." Maybe that is what is causing the nausea.

Friday, June 10, 2005

The last day of radiation!!!!! John got up at around 7:30 hungry! He fed himself a can of Boost. About half an hour later he injected his meds. He also had a couple of sips of water through his mouth. That is the first time anything has gone through his mouth since last Sunday when he had some leftover mashed potatoes.

Something else he learned today from the other doctor on this study, Dr. Greene, was he could use flat root beer to thin out the mucus in his mouth. Another trick is to dissolve a small amount of Adolph's Meat Tenderizer in water and swish that around in his mouth. Learn something new every day.

John's supervisor, Captain Lawrence, stopped by this afternoon after we returned from the hospital. He is really very nice and willing to do anything he can to help John. He even said had he known John wanted his trailer here from Valdosta, he would have rented a truck and brought it with him.

This will probably be the last email until after we get home next week. If anything unusual happens I'll be sure to let you know. My apologies for this being so very long. I guess I had diarrhea of the mouth (fingers?) this time. Please pray that John feels well enough to travel next Tuesday.

Love, Affection and Blessings

K

Saturday, June 11, 2005

While John was getting fluids yesterday, he received a phone call from the Patient Squadron informing him he had a meeting with someone named Dona at the Medical Evaluation Board (MEB). Dona informed him that his case would be going to the MEB probably Tuesday or Thursday of next week. They will make the determination as to his duty status. There are several decisions they can make. He can be returned to active duty (but not on flying status) while still undergoing treatment; he can be temporarily medically retired; or he can be permanently medically retired.

Based on what she said, I had the sense that she was not holding out much hope for John to be maintained on active-duty status.

One of the things I have learned about cancer patients is a large part of their battle is maintaining a positive attitude and outlook. I know this Dona cannot possibly be aware of John's situation but even if she was, I am not sure she would have or could have approached what she had to say any differently.

John has had several goals throughout this whole ordeal. The first is to beat this cancer as quickly as possible, then to be near to his children who are in Valdosta. Next is returning to flying status and last is to stay in the service at least until he has reached 20 years which will be next March 21st. What John heard, as did I, was: He can forget about returning to flying, that's not going to happen. He probably won't be able to make his 20 years and he will not be returning to Moody AFB in Valdosta. Her actual words were "Well, we all know that dog ain't gonna hunt!" You could just see John deflate. He seemed to shrink before my eyes. John was totally devastated. I could not believe she said that to him! I was speechless.

Dona referred to herself as his advocate. Ha! I seriously don't believe she even knows what the word means! Dona is supposed to understand what he wants and then fight for him to get it. The process of doing the evaluation and any appeals John might want to use if the determination is not to his liking, would probably be no longer than three months, which would put it at about the time his treatment is over. So, he has to do all this while he is undergoing chemotherapy. If he does not agree with the first determination, he can appeal through a special board right here in San Antonio. If that does not give him the answer he wants, the next and last appeal is to the Secretary of the Air Force. The Air Force would provide a lawyer whose expertise is in medical law. Can you imagine getting chemotherapy treatment and having to come up with a written appeal and also preparing to "testify" to a group of people on why you should be kept on active duty? I'd like to see a corporation try to do something like this to an employee under the same circumstances. How a determination of this magnitude can be made in the middle of his treatment is more than I can understand.

He was feeling better yesterday before he heard this news, but now he is feeling really bummed out. With everything he has gone through in the past few years, to have this thrust upon him in the manner that it was, is just about too much. We'll just have to wait and see how he does this next week or so.

Wednesday, June 15, 2005

Wow!! What a weekend and early week we had this week. Almost all day Saturday and Sunday John spent in bed. I think it was a combination of the relief of the radiation being over as well as just feeling rotten because of the radiation and the news he heard from Dona.

On Monday morning we went to the hospital so John could get more fluids. Before we did that, we went to the patient squadron and spoke with Karen. John told her what had happened and she said the only way the MEB could have gotten started was because the doctor had written them the narrative, which she had. Karen had spoken with the doctor for some paperwork, but that was in connection with his transfer to Lackland. We left Karen and went down for fluids and I went to see Maggie.

When I told her what we had been told on Friday she said she would look into it for us. She called Dona and within one hour Dona was downstairs in the chemo room where John was, all apologetic. She could not believe she had left us with the impression that John was going to be put on a medical retirement. Dona said she "was just giving us the worst case." Unfortunately, no-where in the conversation on Friday did she say this was the worst case. She was so upset she was even in tears.

Once we heard that this was the case, John began to perk up somewhat. Later that afternoon we had a meeting with the chemo oncologist, Dr. Gallagher and she confirmed she had sent the narrative to the MEB. She indicated she would not have done that unless she had been asked. John asked her who had requested it and she said it was Karen. Now you know what the communication is like in the military. It is like that old game where someone makes a statement, whispers it to the person next to them, and by the time it gets around the room, it is nothing like what was originally said. So, this all started because of a misunderstanding about what was being requested.

On Monday afternoon we went to notify the front desk that we were checking out on Tuesday and asked for a late checkout. They have no policy for a late checkout so we had to pay for an extra day to stay beyond noon. OK. Did that. John was now hungry and suggested we go out for dinner! Please understand John had nothing go down his throat from Sunday the 5th of June until Monday the 13th when he had some water. He was hungry enough he wanted to try some mashed potatoes. Since we had gotten rid of all the food except something he could not eat, this is what he decided he wanted to do. We decided we would get the rest of the packing done first, then go.

By the time we did finish, he was about finished as well. So, I wound up going to Popeye's Chicken and getting him some mashed potatoes. When I brought them home, we loaded them up with butter and cheese and he was able to eat the whole order.

Tuesday morning, we went back to the hospital and he got fluids. He now weighed 197. Everyone was remarking on how well he had done. He had lost about 15 pounds total even without eating much. And the people in the radiation department were impressed with the fact that he took all 33 radiation treatments without asking for a break. That was really rough on him, but he would not admit it. Anyway, we came back home and finished the last-minute stuff, finished the checkout process, and John decided to lay down for a nap. Just before he did, the housekeeper knocked and said she was sure she had seen us walk into the apartment but her supervisor said we were gone because we were checked out. We told her we would be leaving about 2:30 or 3:00.

John went in for a nap and a few minutes later, the phone rang. It was the front desk calling to ask why we were still there when we had checked out. In the rudest tone possible I heard, "Well, you are just going to have to pay for an additional day and have an inspection." When I told her we had already done that the day before, she said she would have to speak to her supervisor. Fine. I found the bill which I did not have at my fingertips when I spoke with her and called her back. When I explained what I was looking at she said, "Wait just a minute while I look that up." Now why couldn't she have done that BEFORE she called me in such a snit? I'm telling you that front desk needs a LOT of work.

About five minutes later the phone rings again, but this time it is John's Commanding Officer. This time I woke John and they talked for some time. When they finished John came out of the bedroom and told me he had some bad news. I am not sure if I told you about his 1st Sgt.'s mother sending John some cookies when we first got there but she did. Anyway his 1st Sgt. is coming to Lackland from Iceland next week because they found an abnormality in his lung area. John really feels bad about that.

Then he told me some good news. His CO really called to tell him that he was being promoted to Master Sergeant. John was really pumped. He said he couldn't tell anyone in the military until the 16th then proceeded to get on the phone to tell a few of his close friends. I tell you that news and the fact that he was going to see his boys that evening made all the difference. His voice got stronger and he was antsy to get moving to the airport. So, we did.

I dropped him at the airport while I went to turn in the rental car. When I got back to the airport, he had already checked in for both of us. We left there around 9:45 pm and arrived in Cincinnati at 1:00 am. His boys were at the airport and absolutely thrilled to see him as he was to see them. By the time we got our luggage and arrived home it was 2:00 and we went to bed around 3:00.

Today he looked really good, messed around with his truck a bit then took a nap. Me, I went to get a pedicure, a new set of nails and my hair done. Can't beat that for a gorgeous spring day.

Friday, June 17, 2005

Yesterday not much happened. John mostly worked on his truck and took naps. Had to get to bed really early because of his appointment with the doctor at Wright Pat. I was going to go with him along with Ray but had a problem with my computer and had to stay home to get it fixed. That could be another book but I won't go into it here.

The doctor said John was doing fine. They did blood work and all his levels are great. He does have an infection at the peg. On Thursday night he was trying to feed himself through the peg and something started to fall. When he tried to get it, he jerked on the tube and pulled it. He was in real pain for a few minutes. That is where the infection is, so the doctor gave him some antibiotics and circled the red spot. If, 24 hours after he started the antibiotics the redness has not diminished, he is to call the doctor.

He is attempting to eat small amounts of food more often now and is doing very well with that. And he is drinking more and more water. For now, all the news is good. At least for John.

My washing machine is leaving large black, grease-like spots on our clothes and the dryer sounds as though it is on its last legs. So as soon as I get this mailed, Ray and I are out looking for replacements.

Love, Affection and Blessings

K

Monday, June 20, 2005

The truck is finally fixed!!!! John and Ray have spent almost all their spare time working on it and today John finished. Ray had to work this morning.

We had sort of a quiet weekend. John took his seed to a movie one night then they went with Marjorie, her children, and Roxanne and her children to play putt-putt golf another day. (Tracy was working and Stephanie had gone to Detroit to visit her fiancé, Chris.) Then on Sunday after church, everyone came here to celebrate Father's Day. The day was the usual wildness with seven grandchildren. The other three were on their own adventures.

Vacation Bible School started today at our church and I had told Roxanne I would be there to help out. Trent, John's youngest, got up on the wrong side of the bed today so I told him he had to promise me he would not have a good time. Well, he did have a good time in spite of himself. He just wants to sleep in a bit later so he says.

For some unknown reason, John was unable to eat or drink anything today. I'm thinking maybe something he ate yesterday was too rough and perhaps he irritated his throat.

Thursday, June 23, 2005

John and Ray went to Wright Pat again yesterday. The doctor looked at his throat but did not comment other than to say it looked a bit raw. He received more fluids and it is a good thing because he still is not able to even drink water. And I know he does not inject enough water through the tube. He is still on Percoset, Triple Mix (but he doesn't use it because he cannot swallow anything), pain patches and antibiotics.

I said the truck was fixed on Monday. Wrong!!!! Something was wrong with the brakes when John went to leave last night to visit a friend of his. Had to turn around and come back home. Hopefully, it will get fixed tomorrow. Boy, is Ray going to have a great time on the road in this truck! It does have well over 200,000 miles on it.

John and Ray took Trent to the airport today. He was supposed to be going home tomorrow but there was a change in plans and he had to leave today. I think it was a bit hard for John to say goodbye.

Saturday, June 25, 2005

I'll tell you what, I am very glad this week is over. It was fun seeing the Dominoes group, people from church and attending a Zonta meeting but I am exhausted mainly from Vacation Bible School. I am going to need this next week to recuperate.

Let me tell you about my adventure on Thursday night on the way to the meeting. I picked up a friend of mine and we are tooling down I-71 just about keeping up with traffic when I look at the speedometer. "Oh my God, Jean! I know I am not traveling 101 miles per hour but look at the speedometer." Then I looked at the odometer and it read 48,800 miles. Earlier in the day I remembered it was 30,200. This is a leased car so I try to keep track of the miles driven.

All of the readings were totally messed up. As soon as we got to the meeting place, I called Ray and told him. He said we would have to take the car in the next day. That being impossible for me, I said he would have to do it.

After the meeting, on the way home, I remarked to Jean that the temperature had dropped two degrees. It had read 33 on the way to the meeting and now read 31. Then I saw it. Next to the 31 was a very small "c." I asked Jean to be sure and she confirmed what I saw. Then I looked at the speedometer and saw the small "km."

There is a button on the dashboard which can be changed from the normal readings to the English metric system. I must have inadvertently pushed that button. Sure made me feel stupid but relieved at the same time. Could you just see Ray taking the car into the dealer complaining about the computer system and it be nothing more than pushing a button? He would have been a bit peeved if he had not seen it first himself.

Everyone was here yesterday except Tracy for dinner. She had to work. They all came to say goodbye to John and Dean. John still is not able to eat or drink anything.

After everyone left last night, Dean found Bret's wallet downstairs. Called Marjorie and told her and while on the phone Dean realized he left his military ID at Marjorie's house. So today when the three of them left here, (John, Dean, and Ray) they had to stop at Marjorie's to exchange "stuff." They left there around 10:30.

My mother and I went to Kroger as they were having a sale on things she uses all the time. When we got back there was a message from Ray asking me to call him back. Please, God, not an accident.

No, not an accident. Do I know where John has put the keys to the trailer? Now, tell me, how am I supposed to know that? No, I don't know. John got on the phone and directed me to his motorcycle. Open this compartment and that compartment. No keys. After searching the house for about half an hour, I called them back. John tells me he usually keeps them in the truck, but they are not there. He has some keys which will allow him to enter a small compartment on the outside of the trailer and perhaps the keys are there but he doubts it. Oh well, a locksmith will be needed, maybe.

I don't know what I would have done this week without Roxanne. She had the only usable washing machine in the family. Marjorie is unable to use hers because of a sewer problem and Tracy's is on its last legs and, of course, mine had two legs on a banana peel and two legs in the appliance graveyard. I ordered a new one last Friday and was told it should be here this Friday. Of course, it is not and now they don't think it will be in until early next week. Because I was tied up with VBS and an assortment of other appointments, Marjorie, who I think was supposed to be on vacation this week, took clothes to Roxanne's house and did them. I only sent the clothes of the male members of this household. At least they could take clean clothes on this trip. I just hope the new washing machine arrives before I leave next Sunday.

I intend to do nothing for the rest of the day and probably tomorrow.

Love, Affection and Blessings

K

Monday, June 27, 2005

Ray and John are finally on their way to San Antonio, but not without yet another problem. They did manage to get into the trailer last night, but without keys. They were not where John thought they might be. There is a trap door under the trailer and John crawled through that. After they were in, they discovered mice. I am sooo looking forward to living in that thing for three months. NOT!!!!!! John assures me the mice will be gone before I get to San Antonio. Uh-huh.

They did not sleep in the trailer last night. A friend in Lakeland, which is about 35 miles northeast of Valdosta, invited them to spend the night. What with the mice and all it might have been just a bit too crowded for Ray and John in the trailer.

They did get a locksmith to make new keys for the trailer today. I guess once they got everything ready to go, they discovered the battery was dead. So, there was one more delay. Ray called about 5:00 pm and they were waiting on the battery then they were going to head out. It was my understanding that John wanted to go to Crestview FL to check on his house there and to renew his driver's license before heading west. I don't know if that was still part of the plan with all the other delays. Ray said he would call when they stopped tonight. It is now 9:00 PM and they have yet to call so they may have decided to get as far as they can tonight before stopping.

Ray did say that other than being a bit tired, John seems to be doing well. Ray is making him stop every hour and a half to inject either water or Boost, to keep his fluid levels up. I guess he still cannot eat. Ray said he, Ray, has only eaten one meal today so he may be losing some weight on this trip as well. Not that he couldn't afford to lose some.

John's daughter, Gemma is coming here on the 29th to spend a few days with her cousins before we head to Texas. She will be flying from England to Orlando, then on the same day getting on another plane and coming here. They made the reservations to Orlando before knowing she would be coming here. I guess it would cost too much to change the reservation at this late date. The reason for Orlando is her mother and brothers are going to be at Disney World this week.

Wednesday, June 29, 2005

I phoned Ray about 7:00 pm last night and they were 60 miles from San Antonio. I really could not believe it. Pulling a 32-foot trailer they made it in just over one day. On Monday at around 5:00 pm they were not yet to Pensacola and they stopped in a rest area and slept until 5:00 am yesterday. At 10:00 pm here Ray phoned to say they were on the base, at the campsite, under a tree, hooked up to electricity and water and John was already in bed. That's a lot of driving. I guess the trip took more out of John than he thought it would.

I think that being under a tree is nice but I have heard there are scorpions out there and some of them are in trees. Let's see, mice, scorpions, hmmm. I am so very excited to get there I am about jumping out of my skin.

Last night there was a storm early in the evening and about 10:00 the electricity started going off and on about four times. About 11:00 it went off for good. I don't know what was going on but was thinking wouldn't it be just my luck to have the washer and dryer delivered tomorrow and then have no electricity? Service was restored at about midnight.

This morning there was just a small bit of excitement. I had just gotten out of the shower when the security alarm went off. My mother forgot it was on and opened the door. I turned it off and within one minute the phone rang. It was the security people. "What is your name and your password? Is everything alright?" Nice to know they are on top of things.

Love, Affection and Blessings.

K

Friday, July 01, 2005

John had an appointment with the Chemo oncologist, Dr. Gallagher yesterday. Since he left there on June 14th he has lost nine pounds. He is now down to 190. That was his secret ambition anyway to reach that weight. Now we will have to see if he keeps it on. He is still not eating but they are not worried about that too much since he is using the Boost. Dr. Gallagher said that it would be three to four weeks after his last radiation treatment before he would be able to eat anything. I think we were hopeful it would be sooner since he was eating little bits when we first came home.

Maggie called me at home today looking for John. She left a message saying she had tried to call his cell number but no one answered.

And of course, you cannot leave a message on his cell. I called Ray and told him to call her right away as she was leaving the hospital very soon. Today is a holiday for them as well as Monday. Turns out all she wanted was to know how he was feeling.

While at the doctor's office, John said he mentioned to Maggie that he was still having some trouble with constipation. I asked if he was using the Senecot and he said he was out of it. How about going to the drugstore and buying some more???? How hard is that? John said she gave him some medication that he could not swallow. But he said it is a liquid gel capsule. When Ray got on the phone again, he said they were going to break all of them open and have John inject all at once. I pleaded with them to please do this before I got there!!!!! I think he was only kidding.

Ray told me the other day that there was a leak in the trailer. One more something to look forward to. Then today I spoke with Carole, Ann's sister-in-law and she told me there had been absolutely no rain and it was sooo very hot. So how did they know there was a leak you might ask, as did I?

Well, John climbed up onto the roof and told me it "was soft," whatever that means. I asked him, since it was still under warranty if he had found anyone there who would honor the warranty and fix it. "No, I haven't even started to look. I figured I might just leave it and wait until I get it back to Valdosta and take it back to the dealer and have them fix it."

"So, what are you going to do if it rains in the meantime? And just exactly where is this leak?"

"Well, the soft spot is in the back of the trailer and there are some water marks inside the trailer. If it rains, I guess I'll just put a tarp over the top of it."

Now then, the back of the trailer is the second bedroom. Guess where I am supposed to sleep when I get there? And a tarp over the top! This just keeps getting better and better.

Monday, July 04, 2005

Greetings from San Antonio! Happy Independence Day!

I don't think I mentioned before that John's daughter Gemma had come to Cincinnati on the 29th and she and I were flying to San Antonio together on Sunday July 3rd. She spent most of her time in Cincinnati with her cousins and on Saturday she came over to our house with Tracy. Tracy is staying at our house again to be with my mother while we are gone.

Gemma had asked her dad if it was ok if she came to San Antonio after her family got home from Disney World which would have been after the 5th of July. Of course, he said sure. She told him she was not sure if she could make it or not because she did not know for sure what her schedule was going to be. Then she called Marjorie and asked if she could come to Cincinnati first and then fly to San Antonio on the 3rd to surprise her dad. I was afraid Ray would spill the beans but I guess he didn't.

We arrived in San Antonio yesterday without a problem. I had reserved a car with Hertz so we took the shuttle to the Hertz lot. Since I had already reserved the car, I only needed to show them my credit card because I rented it on a multi-month contract. I told Gemma just to wait with the luggage and I would be right out. Well, the people ahead of me did not understand what was going on when they were asked for a credit card. Long story short, 30 minutes later I finally got waited on. Poor Gemma had been waiting in the heat all this time. And it was HOT. We got into this thing they call a car, and proceeded to the base. This car was a Kia with no automatic windows, no automatic door locks and the right-side view mirror could not be adjusted from the driver's seat.

Well, when we got to the trailer, Ray was sitting outside and John was inside watching the ball game. Gemma got out of the car and went to the door. John came out and was just about speechless. He was truly surprised. He did not think he could be had, but he was. He even said that now he knows how it feels.

We went out to eat last night and, of course, John just sat and watched. I guess it is really getting to him that he just cannot swallow. Not even his own saliva. When we got home, we were pretty tired so we just crawled into bed.

John looks pretty good considering he has lost nine pounds since he was home in Cincinnati. He is taking about six cans of Boost plus six bottles of water each day.

Tomorrow John starts chemo. He said he will be getting one dose of Cisplatin then a continuous infusion of Fluorouracil otherwise known as 5FU for four days. I guess they will give him some sort of bag to carry with him. He will have to go to the hospital every day for those four days to get fluids. The Cisplatin that he will receive will be a lower dose than what he received during radiation. The 5FU is not supposed to give him the nauseous feeling he experienced before. Let's pray the hiccups are a thing of the past.

Tuesday, July 05, 2005

Last night the fireworks display was really pretty good. Not anything close to Riverfest, but good. Actually, there were two different displays: one behind us from another base, I think Kelly, and the one on the side of us from right here on Lackland.

This morning John had to be at the hospital at 9:30. The first thing they did was an EKG. Then they gave him a new medication called Emend. This is yet another anti-nausea medication. It is different from the others in that it is taken along with the others not instead of the others. It has one pill of 125 MG to be taken on the first day one hour before the treatment, and two other 80 MG pills to be taken on days two and three after the treatment.

He was very weak again today and very tired. He took a nap yesterday, but not a long one. I hope he can sleep while getting the treatment so he gains some strength. He also looks longingly at the food we are eating or at the TV when they are advertising things he would like to eat. Perhaps that will motivate him to try to eat something, although I saw Maggie today at the hospital and she said it may last for a while longer.

He seems to be hacking and coughing more and more these days. He still wakes up a lot during the night.

Ray and I left him at the hospital this morning because there is so much to do back here at the trailer. It is rather cool this morning so hopefully we can get done what needs to be done while it is still cool. Ray is even going to go do the laundry. Sheets and towel, only! Many years ago, he tried to do some laundry for me and put bleach in colored clothes. Never again!

When Ray went to get John this afternoon, he was sound asleep. The bag they gave John for the 5FU is put into a box that measures how much he is getting. That box is then put into a fanny pack. This one bag of 5FU lasts for 96 hours. It is attached to a tube which goes into his port.

They gave him a schedule for the month of August, but not for July. We do know he meets with the radiation oncologist next week and the chemo oncologist the week after. He also has some lab work done around the 18th. Even though he only gets this treatment for four days in a month, he is kept pretty busy with other appointments.

While he was getting the treatment today, I took Gemma shopping for shorts. A new Wal*Mart just opened near the base and she wanted to go there to get some more shorts. While out, I decided even if John got upset, I was going to buy some things that were going to make my life easier. Like an ironing board. Not a full-size one, but one that sits on a table. Also, a couple of casserole dishes. He has no glass dishes. So, anything that goes into the microwave has to be put into a plastic dish or bowl. Not anymore!

When we got home, I decided I would start to clean out some cabinets. Now Ray had already cleaned the cabinets as in washing them. What neither he nor John did was to look at the expiration date on a lot of stuff. I got rid of four or five plastic bags full of stuff. You would be surprised at how much more room there is now in the cabinets. I tried to show John what I had done so he wouldn't be looking for something and wonder where in the world I put it. "Ma, I'm not worried about it. Whatever you did is fine." Wish he was always so pliable. Tomorrow, I start on the closets and try to make some room for my clothes. John has heavy clothes in his closets and with the weather being at 100°F, I don't think he will be using them for a long while.

Wednesday, July 06, 2005

When John got up this morning his face looked like he had a sunburn. The burn from the radiation had diminished a lot before this. As a matter of fact, the scabbing had completely gone by the time Gemma and I arrived in San Antonio. That's why it was a surprise to see his face so red and only from just below the eyes down. I asked the doctor when she stopped in while John was getting fluids and she explained that at times the chemo will cause a throwback to the effects of the radiation. I just wonder if that is also going to have an effect on his throat and not allow him to eat for a longer period of time.

He found out today that his orders have been cut to have him PCS'd to Lackland. The only thing is the orders are not here yet. So, for the time being, he is still on Temporary Duty status. Also, he has not heard anything as yet from the MEB but I am sure that will come shortly.

They gave him two new medications today in addition to the three for nausea. There is yet one more he is supposed to take. One is called Lorazepam (Ativan). He doesn't think he will need to take that. The other prescription Dr. Gallagher gave him is for Loperamide (Imodium) which is supposed to be for loose stools. Considering he had trouble with hard stools, this seems to be a bit off. I know he is not going to take this one.

When I went to pick up his prescriptions, I asked about having mine filled. I was told I could not because they were not from a doctor here in Texas. So much for being prepared. I am going to ask John's doctor if she will write prescriptions for me so I can get my own meds.

Love, Affection and Blessings

K

Thursday, July 7, 2005

I stayed home this morning to do some laundry while Ray took John over to the hospital. Gemma was allowed to sleep in. I had a couple of phone calls to make and before I knew it Ray was back. I finally got the laundry started about 11:00 AM.

We got one of the closets empty of John's winter jackets and I did the ironing. Later, after John got back home and took a nap, we went to the other side of the base so he could sign the necessary paperwork to extend until 2007. Because he got the promotion, he is required to commit to another two years. What a chore that turned out to be. I thought this was going to be a five or ten minute deal so I stayed in the car. About 20 minutes later Gemma came out and said this was going to take longer than we anticipated so I had better come in because of the heat.

After waiting another ten minutes a Sergeant came over and took over the job of figuring out what to do. It seems that John's situation is just a bit different. Number one, he has not yet PCS'd here; although his orders are in Iceland, they have not yet reached here: Number two, he has some sort of a code behind his name which is confusing to them: Number three, he is an outpatient at Wilford Hall: And number four, his case is going to the Medical Evaluation Board (MEB).

They had to call the Air Force Military Personnel Center (AFMPC) to find out just exactly what he could or could not do. At first, they said he would not be allowed to extend. Then they looked in a manual and found if he was intending to re-enlist, he would not be allowed to do that because of the MEB. After the phone call, it was determined he was able to extend but they don't know who has to sign the paperwork; his old Colonel in Iceland, some Colonel here in Lackland, or a Colonel in this hospital. It would appear any old Colonel might do.

While this discussion is going on, another woman enters the scene with a manual in hand. It would seem that a "63" must be filled out. "Why?" says the Sergeant "When all we ever needed was this letter? We have been doing all the extensions and re-enlists with just this letter." Oh well! Times they are a changin'. John is then told he doesn't have to do anything until this "63" has been issued by the AFMPC. These are also the people who told the Sergeant that John could only legally extend for three-month increments but to go ahead and have him extend for the full two years. Supposedly they will deal with all the legalities later.

Sometime today John got a call from Dona. Remember her from the MEB? She was wondering why he had not yet checked in with her. He had told her he would call her when he returned to San Antonio. Unfortunately, (ha) he forgot. We are going to need to stop and see her tomorrow while we are at the hospital.

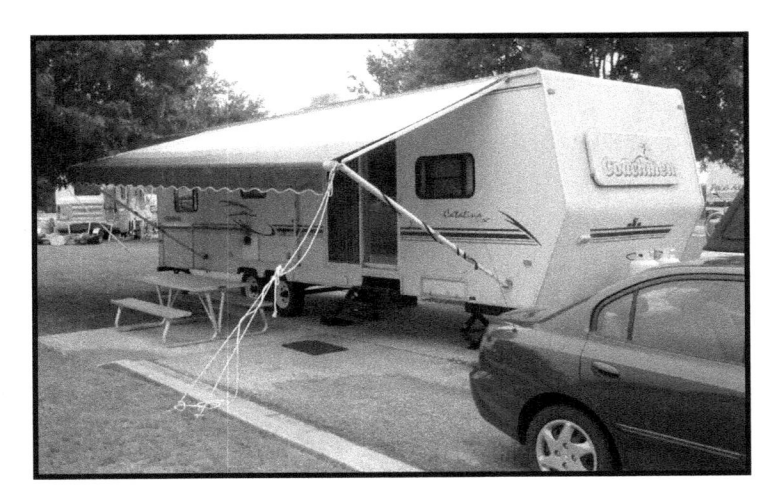

For those of you who have not had the pleasure of the experience, let me tell you a bit about trailer living. First of all, everything is toy-sized. When you enter the trailer, to one's immediate right is a doorway leading to the master bedroom. There is a large bed, one long closet and one short closet. There is enough room to move around the bed if you are careful not to stub your toes or scrape your knees. There is also a shelf under the short closet with a couple of drawers. There is another shelf in front of the long closet on which John has placed a TV. It is also a catch-all station. Over the top of the bed are two small cabinets. There are three windows all of which have mini blinds perpetually closed. There are curtains as well. Under the bed there is a storage unit. All one need do is pull up the mattress.

When you enter the trailer, immediately in front of you is a three-cushion sofa that pulls out to a bed. A lumpy bed, but a bed. To the right is a shelf with a TV on it, a built-in radio with a tape deck, a cd player and a clock. Below the radio, etc. there are two very small shelves, one with a door and one without. Above the TV is a corner cabinet. Across from the TV is a table on a slightly raised platform. There are two benches, one on either side of the table. These benches open up to reveal storage areas. There are three windows with mini-blinds here as well.

Now then, the kitchen. The first thing you notice is a toy stove with three burners. Count em! One, two, three. There is an oven but you cannot fit a cookie sheet into it. You can put a 9x12 pan in there. Over the top of the stove is an exhaust fan with a light. Over this is the microwave shelf with the microwave on it. The switch for the fan and light is recessed to the very back of the top of the exhaust. And of course, the bottom of the microwave shelf extends out over the exhaust by about four inches. It is a real challenge to turn this on or off. Also, even as tall as I am I cannot see into the bowl or cup or whatever is in the microwave without standing on a step stool, which is kept under the table. Under the oven is the hot water heater.

Next to the stove is a counter space of about five inches total and next to that is a double sink. Picture a giant-sized postage stamp and you have the size of this double sink. Next to this is another five-inch countertop. There is more room behind the sink which of course is taken up with a set of bowls that do not fit into any of the cabinets or the dish drainer. Over the top of the sink is one double-door cabinet and another single-door cabinet on the side wall. The double cabinet has two shelves but only one in the single door. Below the sink is the most cabinet space with the exception of the back bedroom

There are three small drawers and when I say small, I mean small. There is one large drawer that is only half as deep as the small drawers but twice as wide. You cannot fit any paper product in it such as waxed paper, Saran Wrap or aluminum foil. The only thing that will fit are small baggies.

There is a large cabinet where all the cleaning supplies are supposed to go plus the paper products. Next to that is a very small triangular cabinet. Next to that is the door leading to the bathroom and next to the door, facing the sink is a refrigerator and freezer. There are half sized shelves in this refrigerator and two very small vegetable bins. The freezer is a top side, she said laughingly. You can put a few things in there but not much else. Looks as though I will be shopping on a more regular basis that I am used to.

When John is standing at the sink feeding himself through the tube, and Ray is next to him helping, don't try to open the door to either the refrigerator or the bathroom or you will knock into either or both of them.

Enter the bathroom. Teensy teensy tiny shower. Don't try to turn around, but then you ARE standing in the tub so should you not like getting knocked in the head with the shower head, you could sit down to bathe. When you do take a shower, you cannot let the water run as I am used to doing. If I do that we will run out of hot water. The shower head is equipped with an on/off switch. You don't have to reset the temperature each time so that is a plus. Opposite the shower is the sink which is considerably smaller than the kitchen sink. There is a counter to the left of the sink with another shelf underneath. There is also a cabinet but a lot of the room in there is taken up by the plumbing. (The same is true of the cabinet under the kitchen sink.) Over the top of the sink and the shelf is a cabinet with two shelves each about two inches deep. Well, maybe three inches. It does go from the kitchen wall to the bedroom wall however. Whoa Buddy! The commode is similar to one I have seen on a boat. The flush has a handle but it works in the most unusual way. I don't even think I can describe this one. Anyway, this fixture is just in front of the open shelf on an angle.

Now we enter the back bedroom. There is a folding door that clips shut if someone is sleeping there. There are two steps up but please don't try to stand up on the top step as your head will go right through the top of the trailer. Straight ahead is a cabinet of sorts. It is really a chifforobe with two large (you get the picture when I say large; everything is relative) drawers. On either side of this storage facility is a bunk bed. Currently Gemma is sleeping on one of them and the other is used for storage as is the area underneath the beds. And we do have a bunch of stuff to store!!!!!!

Ray has been doing little odd jobs to keep busy. But there is just so much that can be or needs to be done. He has fixed Gemma's suitcase. The handle had come loose. He worked on the truck a bit but said he couldn't get to the area he needed to get to. He fixed the screen door on the trailer and leveled it a bit more so the water would run off the front of the trailer instead of the back. He also repositioned the awning so if a gust of wind comes along it won't take the awning with it.

Sunday, July 10, 2005

On Friday we saw Maggie while waiting for John to get fluids at the hospital. We said he still could not swallow then he told her it felt as though someone was choking him all the time. She seemed puzzled by that and said that she would tell Dr. Peterson about it. John said at one time that he was afraid to try to swallow. He also told me that the left side of his tongue is really sore. I know nothing he has tried has helped the mucositis. Not even the really expensive Gelclair.

Just after John went in to get his fluids, I received a phone call from the people at the personnel office we had visited on Thursday. The "63" was ready for John's signature so as soon as he was finished with getting his fluids we went over there. He signed the form then was informed he would have to take an oath. The problem was there was no one in their department who was an officer to administer the oath. The sergeant went all over the building looking for one and finally found one on the second floor. So now that he has been officially sworn in, the paperwork gets faxed to Iceland for his commanding officer's signature then faxed back here. That is to be done on Monday.

I also ran into Dona in the hallway on Friday morning and she said John does not need to come to her office unless there is something he wanted to change on the narrative Dr. Gallagher wrote. The only thing on there that was in error was that he had received antibiotics in Iceland. The MEB meets on Tuesday. I am not sure what happens after that.

On Saturday John had to be at the hospital to get de-accessed at 8:00 AM. Ray went with him this time instead of me. John has been so tired lately that all he wants to do is sleep. As soon as he got home, he went to bed and slept for the better part of the day. He seemed to feel much better when he got up.

John had the beginnings of Tinnitus early in the treatment. (Tinnitus is a constant ringing in the ear.) I have a slight case of it myself. Now, this session of chemotherapy has exaggerated that so he can hardly hear. Just one more thing he has to deal with.

When Gemma and I arrived here on Sunday there were only a few camp sites in use. Tonight, almost all of them are filled up. Before John and I left here in June I checked here about reservations and regulations. I was told they took no reservations. Maybe I told you this before. Anyhow we might have to leave here for one day if neither the Patient Squadron, Dona, or the person Arnold Fairbanks (our friend's brother) knows can do anything about keeping us here. When they get full, the first person here has to leave for at least a day. I really cannot see breaking camp (see I am even learning the lingo!!!) for one day setting up somewhere else then breaking camp again only to set up here again. Makes no sense to me. But they say you have a two-week limit. Two weeks are up for John on Tuesday.

Monday, July 11, 2005

John did not have a good night last night. He wound up getting sick. Then he was up a lot during the night. This morning he said his stomach really hurt and he felt lightheaded. He is still pretty constipated so we are thinking that may be part of the problem. He went back to bed so we are just waiting to see if he wants to call the doctor when he wakes.

He did not take any Boost this morning. The only kind they had at the hospital last week was vanilla and he really hates vanilla so he said he will take that back today and ask for chocolate. Even though he does not take it through his mouth, he gets a reflux and the taste is pretty awful.

It pains me to think that he may just about start to feel better after being off the chemo for three weeks then it will start again.

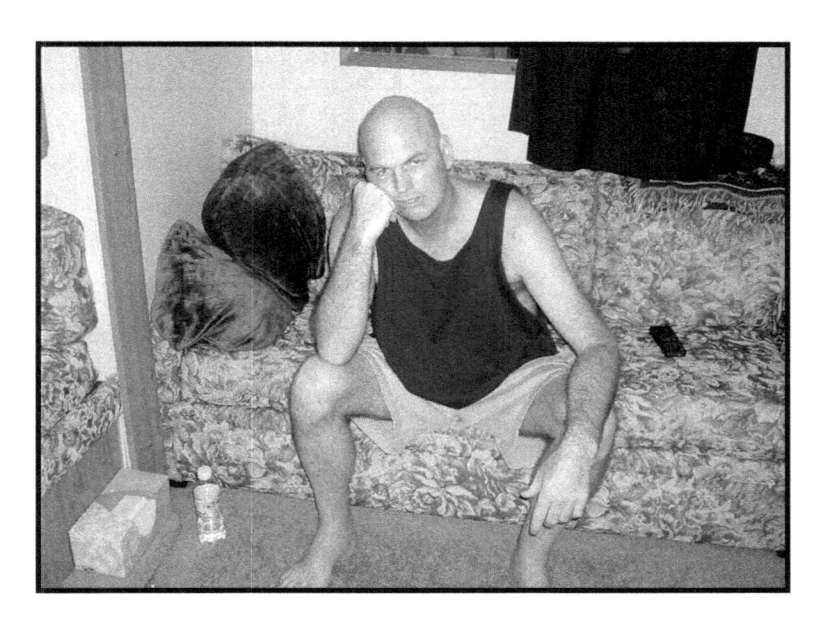

When he woke up he felt somewhat better but not really even 50%. He took some Boost jazzed up with Hershey's syrup. He had to call his commanding officer in Iceland and see Karen at the Patient Squadron among other errands to do so Ray took him to the hospital to do those while I did the laundry. When they got back home, he was going to go right to bed but I guess he felt so bad he decided perhaps he needed some fluids. Ray took him back to the hospital. Ray asked the nurse to call Dr. Gallagher to see if she could come to see him which she did. Dr. Gallagher suggested he take some Senokot and get more fluids tomorrow. He might have one good day to spend with Gemma before she goes home on

Thursday. Ray went to get the Senokot. He is doing the running this week.

Ray is going to go home with Gemma, at least as far as Atlanta. This way he can be sure she gets on the flight to Valdosta ok before he leaves for Cincinnati.

Wednesday, July 13, 2005

This morning Dona called from the MEB. She wants to see John this morning sometime. After we all were up and dressed John and I left. First, we went to the library so he could run copies of letters of recommendation he had received from his commanding officer. Then it was off to see Dona.

The MEB met yesterday and all they do is review all the paperwork submitted by the doctors regarding John's condition. The purpose of our visit there was to review their review, understand what is going to happen next and sign the forms that need to be signed.

The board makes no recommendation, just makes sure all the paperwork is in order. The next step is for Dona to obtain a letter from John's commanding officer, Col. Sanderson stating how John's illness may or may not interfere with him doing his job. In the meantime, John has until Monday at the end of the day to submit his own letter stating why he wants to remain on active duty and why he wants to be returned to Moody AFB in Valdosta, GA when his treatment is over. This is a very important letter for him to write because as I understand it, if he doesn't write this letter, the board will not take into consideration any personal information when determining if he stays on active duty or where he may be stationed.

When we left Dona, we stopped at the Patient Squadron so John could call Iceland using a phone that accepts their DSN number. A DSN number is a prefix similar to an area code but used exclusively by the Air Force going from one Air Force facility to another. It may be used by all the services but at least by the AF.

Karen, at the Patient Squadron, had John's orders finally. He is now officially assigned to Lackland AFB. Of course, it is not as simple as that. She directed us to the Orderly Room in another building to get a checklist. When we arrived there, the person we were supposed to see was at lunch, of course, so someone else took care of John. He was not sure what we were supposed to be getting but he sort of winged it. One of the other clerks there said normally they do not see the patients. When the previous Sergeant in the Patient Squadron was on board, he brought all the paperwork over himself and the patient did not have to be involved at all. Again, times they are a changing!

According to Karen, we are next supposed to go to the Employment Office but not until tomorrow morning. However, the clerk in the Orderly Room said we had to go to Records first. John is by now totally wiped out so we just came back to the trailer. He needs to be at the Employment Office tomorrow morning at 8:00 am. Don't know when we will be going to the Records Office.

John is wanting to take Gemma to Dave and Busters which is a restaurant/arcade. This is in place of going to Fiesta Texas. I just hope he does not over extend himself.

Tomorrow will be a busy day for all of us. First an appointment at 8:00 am then John has an appointment with Dr. Peterson at 10:00 am, then we or I need to get Ray and Gemma to the Airport by 2:30 at the latest. Then a friend of mine is coming in at about 6:30 pm for the weekend.

Thursday, July 14, 2005

John decided to try something to eat last night. Of all things, ice cream. He took a very small amount into his mouth then let it melt some before swallowing. Well, he about doubled over in pain from that. He decided he would take the rest of the ice cream through his peg.

This morning started out on a less than positive note for John. Nothing to do with his in-processing, just that he is in so very much pain. He said it is worse today than it has been before. The pain is because of the mucositis. We were in the employment office and he had to spit into the cup he carries with him and it hurt so badly that for the first time in many, many years, I saw tears coming down his cheeks. I am hopeful that when he sees the doctor this morning at 10:00 he will be able to give him something to take care of the ulcers in his mouth and throat.

The folks in the employment office were going to send him to the finance office today to get his travel vouchers and pay in order. John said absolutely not today. He was in too much pain. When John passes on an opportunity to collect some money, you know he is either feeling really bad or on drugs. In his case it is both!

We saw Dr. Peterson today. When he first came into the room, he wanted to know everything John did since we left for Cincinnati. John could barely talk so I did most of the talking. He did admit, however, that he knew he overdid it with his children, trying to do a lot with them instead of just taking it easy.

The doctor did another scope on him today and I guess that was fairly painful as well. The good news is there is no sign of any tumor in his throat, which I believe, the doctor felt might be a possibility since John is having so much pain when trying to swallow. He does have a severe case of Mucositis. Dr. Peterson said although there are no visible signs of a fungus overgrowth, the possibility of one being there is pretty good. So, for that he prescribed Fluconazole which John was given in May but then in a pill form. This time it is a liquid that he is to intake through the peg for 21 days. Just as an aside, on the bottle there is a label that says: "Discard any used portions after 28 July"

He also told John to increase his Fentanyl patches up to 100 MG at a time. The last time John tried that he got really sick to his stomach so he may only go up to 75. In addition, the doctor prescribed liquid morphine. He didn't like it too much the first time he had it but then it was going in by mouth. This time it will be going in through the peg. That may make a difference.

Love, Affection and Blessings.

K

Sunday, July 17, 2005

Going back to Thursday, I told you a friend of mine, whom I first met in the early 70's at GE and have remained close to all these years came to visit. She wrote back in April that she wanted to come here to give me support but could not until after June. Well, Carolyn arrived on Thursday evening. I prepared a salad with fried chicken and we just ate here. She is claustrophobic and decided she could not stay in the trailer (gee, I can't imagine!) but we were able to get her a room at the Air Force Inn.

On Friday we looked in the phone book for Day Spas and found one that could accommodate both of us around 12:30. What a wonderful treat that was. A one- hour full body massage. I was sooo relaxed when I was finished my legs were weak. When we finished with the massage there was a cute little restaurant on the grounds where we decided to eat. And am I glad we did. The food was wonderful. After lunch, we went outside to the most beautiful rain storm. It had been more than 35 days here in San Antonio without rain so this was welcome. Not only is this a day spa but it is an inn as well. They have three cottages in the back with all kinds of activities on the grounds. There was a huge chess game set up in the garden. This is so large the chess pieces were as big as a kindergartener. They were going to have a small wedding there that evening. All in all, it was a charming place which we thoroughly enjoyed.

We were way on the north side of San Antonio and by the time we got back to the base I was a bit stressed. The sewer system here is not the greatest so a lot of the streets were beginning to flood. Just glad we made it back to the base ok. Later in the evening, I took Carolyn to the North Star Mall where Talbots is. She found a couple of cute outfits between there and Lillian Rubin's. There is also a shoe store here called Clarks that she knew about but I didn't. They were having a sale so of course I found a pair of sandals as did Carolyn. We ate at that same Italian restaurant John and I did when we were there back in May.

On Saturday we went to Riverwalk and to the Alamo. It had rained earlier in the day but when we went, the rain had stopped and the temperature had cooled off considerably. Had lunch at a pretty good Mexican restaurant on Riverwalk, called Mia Casa, I think. We took one of those river tours and the guide was really funny. He was a college student and talked about his plain white polo shirt that was issued by the folks who ran the tours being a "Chick magnet". Then proceeded to flirt with two older women on the river bank to prove his point. Cracked us up.

Came back to the base to check on John but he was doing ok working on his travel voucher so we left again and went to dinner. This time we went to a place that was voted the "best ribs" in San Antonio. We decided we could teach them a thing or two about making ribs.

While we were out running around John stayed close to the bathroom because he has been taking a laxative all week and no results. Today I had to take Carolyn to the airport after a wonderful, wonderful weekend, but John still did not want to leave the trailer. I dropped Carolyn off, then went on to church.

When I came back, SUCCESS, SUCCESS, SUCCESS. John not only felt better, but he looked better. He is even trying to swallow small amounts of liquid. He said he can feel his mouth beginning to heal.

We went to the library but their internet service was down, so we tried the patient library at the hospital but they were closed. We decided to go do a bit of grocery shopping instead. When we got back here, we called the library and the computers were up so back we went.

I did my emailing and responded to some I had received. John came over and said the people in Iceland had closed his email account. He thought he had that fixed to not happen but it happened anyway. The problem with this is he will be unable to get the letters of recommendation that were emailed to him. These letters are to be attached to the letter John is writing to the MEB telling them why he wants to do what he wants to do regarding staying in the Air Force. This, by the way, is called a letter of exception. He is going to go back there tomorrow and call to see if he can get this fixed even on a temporary basis. He is thinking about getting an internet provider so he won't have to depend on the library but I don't know how that would work in the trailer.

When we got back here John was sitting at the table and had a small cup of Aloe Vera Juice which he tipped over. Janie, Mark's wife had emailed me that she gave Mark some of this juice and he is now eating steak! I thought it would be worth a try so John is taking a little at a time. While cleaning up the juice, he knocked over his spit cup. Fortunately, that had mostly mouthwash in it. A few minutes later he was at the sink and started to shake the bottle of Triple Mix. The cap had not been put back on securely and it flew off spilling Triple Mix into the sink. Just after that I was helping him insert some Boost and there was a cup of water sitting on the sink which he knocked over. Butterfingers? Dropsy? What do you think?

Since John's Tinnitus has increased as well as the stuffiness he feels in his head, he has not been able to hear very well. Consequently, the TV is BLARING! Sort of like his dad has the TV volume at home. I sure hope his head clears up soon or I am going to have to spend my time back in the bedroom again.

Speaking of the bedroom, I am now sleeping on the top bunk of the back bedroom. This is a not so wonderful experience as one might think. The first night was not too good as I was constantly thinking I was going to roll off each time I turned. I have sort of gotten used to it now however. It could be I am just too tired to think about it anymore. My feet hit the wall or the chifforobe when I turn. And if I sit up without thinking, I hit my head on the light fixture just over the bed. Ain't life grand?

We still need to clear out the areas under the bunks so we at least know where to find things.

Right now, there is thunder. It has showered a bit today but without thunder. Now thunder. Perhaps we are going to get another good storm. I think probably Tuesday or Wednesday we may get some remains of Emily.

Tonight, John and I worked on his letter of exception to the MEB. He did a pretty good job of getting the information he wanted them to have down on paper.

Monday, July 18, 2005

This morning John is so very much better. He got up early and went to the laundry room to use the phone. Please no, not to do the laundry. He is feeling well enough to drive himself which is a significant improvement. He needed to call Iceland to see if they could retrieve his email and the supporting letters. While he was gone, I decided the bathroom needed to be cleaned. After he returned, he turned around and went to the library. Sure enough there were a couple of letters of recommendation waiting for him. I wish you could read these letters. They are so wonderful. Let me just quote a couple.

"…..I was very impressed with the individual's flight engineer abilities, work ethics, and volunteerism…."

"MSgt. (sel) John Buckler is a superior performer……" "We must retain him and we must find a way to get him back to his assigned duties as an HH-60G Instructor Flight Engineer"

"TSgt. Buckler is a unique commodity in our community….." "Sgt. Buckler has fought back from many adversities and personal issues over the years but not once has he allowed these to interfere with his professionalism and duty performance. Although Sgt. Buckler will not outwardly admit it, his actions have continuously reflected the highest standard of the AF's Core Values."

What a kid!!! I am not too proud, am I?????

While he was at the library, I decided to rearrange the area under the bunk beds. Got that done and decided the sliding glass doors needed to be cleaned. I am just about beat for today.

John returned and showed me the letters. I asked to see the one he wrote. Well, he forgot to print that one. The most important one. I got cleaned up and we went back to the library to run the copies of his letter then headed to the hospital for an appointment with Dr. Gallagher.

She mainly asked questions regarding how he was feeling and what he was not feeling. She said she had asked some people what they knew about the "standard" for returning to flight status from this type of cancer. Well, we already knew there is no standard because this type of cancer is so rare. But the rule of thumb, said Dr. Gallagher is generally five years after the end of the treatment. However, Dr. Gallagher indicated that after one year one can apply for a waiver. John was not too pleased to hear this but she was just telling him what the facts were and he understood.

She talked about him being scheduled for a CT scan this week and suggested that after he met with the ENT physician and after the CT scan, they may look at the possibility of not doing the last chemo treatment. OH MY! Wouldn't that be something? Then she said they really don't recommend doing that because this course of treatment has been successful in saving so many lives, but they also need to look at each case on an individual basis. She said it really hurt her to see John in so much pain as he was last week when she saw him remembering how he was when he first came in to the hospital.

We discussed how this last chemo treatment came on the heels of just returning from the two-week trip to Cincinnati where John admitted he over-extended himself. This next round of chemo, in two weeks, will be after John has done virtually nothing to exert himself so perhaps it will not be nearly as taxing on him as this past one has been.

As I had suspected, the next round of chemo may enhance the side effects John has experienced this time; i.e., the sores in his mouth getting more painful, having more difficulty swallowing, constipation, the tinnitus increasing, etc. I am just praying his being more rested may prove this to be wrong.

When we returned to the trailer, it was about 3:30 and John was tired. I took the laundry and did the wash (six loads) while he took a nap. When I finished, it had poured again. But it stopped long enough for me to get back to the trailer. Then we had a series of thunder storms and it cooled off for a while but got hot and humid all over again.

I don't know if I told you before, but John had ordered another motorcycle while he was in Iceland. He finished paying for it while we were here the first time and it was to have been delivered on the 15th. However, there was a miscommunication and now it won't be here until around the 1st of August. Now then, I have said to John that if he is still on morphine, there is no way he is going to pick up that bike and ride it back to the base. If necessary, says I, I will ride it back to the base. Can you just picture that? Not in his lifetime but any kind of threat will do. I really don't know why another bike, just that it is not nearly as big as the one parked in our garage. I guess this is more for sport riding. I'll keep you posted on who or what brings the bike to the base.

Tuesday, July 19, 2005

Today we both slept in. I didn't get up until nearly 9:45 and John didn't get up until nearly noon. After I showered, I decided to make some chicken noodle soup. I'm thinking pretty soon one of the aromas will trigger a craving in John that he may try to eat something.

Dr. Gallagher called to tell us his appointment is tomorrow at 10:00 for the CT scan. He is to have nothing to eat or drink except water for four hours before the scan.

We are going to go off base today to go to a Target store. On this base there are no rubber scrapers and of course, John has an intense dislike of Wal*Mart so Target it is. Besides, it will be a change of scenery for him. He has not been off the base since last Thursday when we took Ray and Gemma back to the airport.

The aroma of the chicken soup did work today. He said he would like to try a bit of the broth. He ate about two tablespoons and said he would like to try more but he would have to suck up too much morphine and Triple Mix. He decided he would wait a while. But it is a start.

Wednesday, July 20, 2005

This morning John had his appointment to get the CT scan at 10:00. I had a bridge game scheduled so left around 9:20. He had several errands he was going to do today and he was feeling so good he didn't mind if I went out.

His CT scan went on without a hitch. Of course, he will not get the results for some time. He had travel vouchers to file to get reimbursed for his expenses while he has been here. He also had to go to the Patient Squadron and to the library. The travel voucher filing did not go well. It seems when he was first sent here his TDY orders were for 10 days. He was then extended for 70 additional days. He was here for something like 95 days before he was permanently assigned. So now he has to call Lakenheath, England to get that straightened out. They are going to have to amend his orders to reflect the correct length of stay before he can get any money back. And of course, after the call it will take several weeks to get completed.

The rest of the day went ok for him. He did say that when occasionally he says "Ouch" it is because his tongue gets stuck to the roof of his mouth. Evidently the mucus is so sticky that it causes a suction between the roof of his mouth and his tongue. Pulling his tongue off hurts. I tell you I don't know if I would be able to endure the pain he is putting up with.

When you think about it there is almost nothing that has been easy for John since he arrived here. One thing after another seems to go wrong for him. By this time if it were me, I would be tearing my hair out. First, his phone didn't work right and consequently he missed a lot of calls. Then what he heard initially from the woman at the MEB, then he had trouble getting the new bike paid for, then the delivery date got put back, then hearing about the five-year wait or trying to get a waiver to fly earlier, then he is still not getting his mail forwarded from Iceland (sent in two change of address notices plus his friend Chris put one in for him), now the travel vouchers. I know there have been more glitches but I just cannot think of what they were or are. But he takes it all in stride saying "I'm not worried about it."

John took photos of the trailer today. In one of the photos he took, I am asleep on the sofa. (My usual nappy-poo that I take at home when the news is on.) I had no idea he was taking pictures or I would have at least sat up and looked as though I was alert. If you saw these you might get an idea of the area we are living in. You might think the area under the bunk beds still needs to be cleared out. Not so. Already cleared out. What is left is what we need to use but no place to put, so it just stays under the bunk. At least we know where the things are that we need without opening up everything we have.

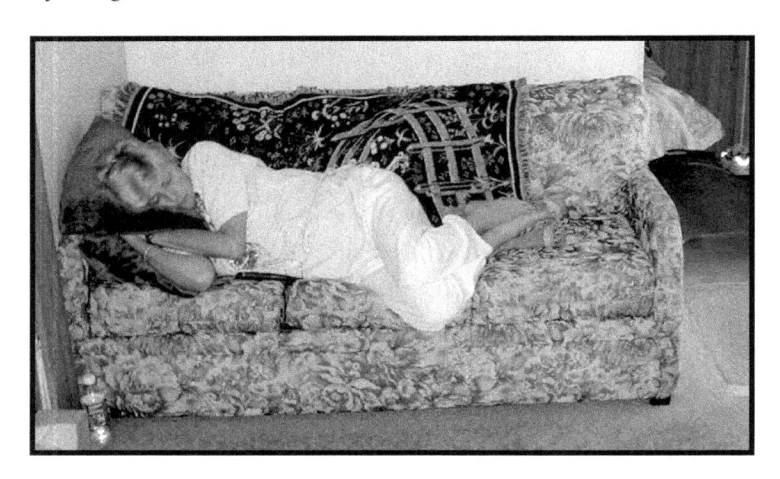

Thursday, July 21, 2005

John got up and left early today to, I thought, call Lakenheath. But then what do I know? Actually, he went to the Patient's Squadron and talked with Karen. She emailed a request to Lakenheath for an amendment to his orders. When he came back to the trailer (I really resist saying "home") he wanted to go to the library right away. We were there for two hours. Obviously, they were not busy or we would have been thrown out after 30 minutes. He got a lot of emailing done as did I. I was also able to clean out my inbox a bunch. I am printing all emails I am receiving from everyone concerning John and they will go into the book I am putting together for him. John forgot to bring his spit cup and did extremely well without it. Perhaps he can begin to wean himself off of it.

We had to go to Walgreens again to get more Magnesium Citrate. Also, more Senokot S. No need to explain why. On the way back we stopped at a small store that sells lottery tickets. While Carolyn was here, she and I bought lottery tickets. I bought scratch-offs and won $13.00. Not too bad.

As soon as we got back John fed himself and went to bed for a nap. He did not take a nap yesterday so was pretty tired today. I have been watching the news about the second round of bombings in London. Sounds like a dastardly deed gone awry (thank God) or some amateur copycats. Either way, enough already!

About 3:30 this afternoon the remnants of Emily came through Lackland. John was still napping but woke with the thunder. He was trying to decide what to do with the awning, when the wind came up with gusto. There is John on one end of the awning and there I am on the other getting soaked in the driving rain while holding down the awning so it won't fly off taking some of the trailer with it. We spent about 15 minutes out there getting absolutely soaked. We saved the awning and the trailer. With the kind of wind we just had, perhaps it was a good thing I was outside. It did get a bit scary when the lightning started, however. When the winds died down, we came in dried off and changed clothes. I don't know if I was glad to be outside the trailer during the wind or not. The slightest bit of wind and the trailer does rock a bit. Oooh, isn't this just ducky? I could have been a-rockin & a-rollin instead of just getting wet in the thunder and lightning!!! About an hour later the rain stopped. It has cooled off so much that we have the door open and John is outside cleaning off part of the trailer that I had suggested needed cleaning while Ray was still here.

John has decided he is going to try some of the chicken noodle soup tonight for dinner including some noodles and chicken instead of just the Boost. Sure hope it goes down ok.

Love, Affection and Blessings

K

Friday, July 22, 2005

Today John had another procedure he was not expecting. He had an appointment with the Ear Nose and Throat doctor because of the feeling of being choked, the sensation of having a stuffy head and some hearing loss.

Last Friday Dr. Peterson spoke by phone to the ENT MD, Dr. Warren, to explain what was going on. Today when John was taken into the exam room a different doctor showed up whom we found out later was in her 3rd week of the 1st year of residency. John's condition was so very far over her head. We asked where Dr. Warren was and were told he had an emergency. This new doctor decided she needed to call in another physician which she did.

Dr. Paul came in and John recognized him and the doctor recognized John. He told us he had reviewed the CT scan and it all looked normal. Thank you, God! Then he said that part of John's problem was the Eustachian tube had shrunk somewhat because of the radiation so fluid was collecting in the middle ear behind the ear drum. This is what was causing the feeling of stuffiness and his hearing everyone as though they were talking in a tunnel.

The answer to this would be to put tubes into John's ears. He said the average stay for these tubes is 8-10 months. John agreed. Dr. Paul said he would do it right there in the office today.

He said John would feel some discomfort and minor pain. What an understatement that turned out to be. The first thing is they cleaned the wax out of his ears. There was quite a build-up of wax in his left ear but hardly any in the right ear. Then they took a long tool with some liquid on it and inserted it into one ear. This was to numb the area. And it stung. Next, they took a thin knife-type tool and cut a hole somewhere in his ear. Then they inserted the tube. Then they took a suction tube and sucked out the liquid. Not much liquid but you would think it was a quart. Actually, probably only a teaspoon. During this whole procedure, John is lying in the chair and grimacing as well as coughing because of the drainage from his sinuses. Occasionally there was a groan.

Now all of you who know me well know I cannot stand anything like this. I am trying to keep my mind occupied by making notes of what was being done and what the doctors were saying. It got to the point where all I could do was look away and take deep breaths. The left ear went fairly well compared to the right ear. When they got to the right ear it took three times before they finally got the tube in. By this time John has turned pale. He has had to stop the procedure a couple of times so he could rise up and cough up the drainage. John's comment about the procedure was "Well that was intense."

When they finally finished, John said he could hear much better. That, however, didn't last very long. They put some antibiotic drops into his ear. The doctor said the fluid in the middle ear could have been infected so this was precautionary. After the drops went in, John could no longer hear better than before. He will need to use these drops three times a day for three days.

I asked him if he thought he was able to walk ok. He said yeah, he was fine. I was not so sure I would be steady on my feet.

He also received a new prescription for Lansoprazole. The common name for this is Prevacid. This is a granule-type product that you dissolve in two tablespoons of water. The purpose of this is to stop the reflux. According to this doctor, when John experiences the reflux, it irritates his throat which in turn causes swelling which could be causing John to feel as though he is being choked. I sometimes get confused by the directions on the labels of these medications. In this instance, the directions on the label say to use in the tube. However, the information paper says don't inject through a feeding tube as the granules may clog the tube. Hopefully, John will be able to swallow it.

We left the trailer this morning at 10:30, the procedure was done, then we had to find Dr. Peterson to make sure the Lansoprazole was ok for John to use because of the clinical study, then find Dr. Gallagher to give her a report of what had been done, then go to the pharmacy to get the prescriptions filled, hit the library and the post office. It was 4:30 before we got back here. And I wondered what we would be doing all day when he is not having chemo treatments.

At about 6:15 John's phone rang and it was a friend of his from Iceland who is in the process of getting transferred here to San Antonio but at Randolph Air Force Base which is on the northeast side of San Antonio. We are on the southwest side. Anyway, Bob, his wife Laurie and their two daughters came to visit. They really are a very nice couple and we enjoyed their visit. John and Bob relived some of their experiences and discussed the happenings at Keflavik, Iceland.

After they left, John was hungry and wanted to try some solid food and something other than soup. He decided he would try some mashed potatoes. He did and after adding some of the broth from the soup to thin them a bit, he got them down. Great job. He had some difficulty but he did it.

He has been drinking the Aloe Vera Juice every day. We need to go get more tomorrow.

Monday, July 25, 2005

A most uneventful weekend. On Saturday we only went to the post office and the library. John was feeling tired, I think from the strain of having the tubes put in Friday so he took a nap while I went to the store to get some more Aloe Vera Juice. His constipation had come back again this week but he was still using the Senokot S and he had success while I was at the store.

Sunday, he felt good enough to go to church and to the store afterward. He wanted to get a flat garden hose. He had one and had used it the other day. When he finished, he turned off the hose but not the water. In the heat of the day the water got so warm and the hose so hot, the hose burst.

When things have gone wrong in the trailer, such as the sewer line backing up, some people have suggested I just pretend I am camping. I HATE camping. It is just not my thing. Ray and John love to camp and Ray is a primitive camper. Rarely uses a tent. Loves the fresh air, sunshine, moonlight, bugs and other creepy crawlies. Just not for me.

There is good news today. John's mucositis is getting better. It is not as thick as it was and he doesn't have to use the spit cup as much. He is also getting some relief from the Gelclair now which he did not get before. And he seems to think the Aloe Vera Juice is helping.

He found out that his email was turned off again yesterday. Now it seems he needs to complete a course before they will turn it on again. He had completed this simple course and needed to fax the certificate to someone in Iceland. Of all the silly things.

He went early this morning to do the faxing and when he came back here, we went to the library immediately. His email is now turned back on; in the meantime, he opened a Yahoo account.

After the library, we went to Records to pick up some of his records that were mailed there. Among the records was the last evaluation his immediate supervisor gave him. He got what is referred to as a "firewall five" rating. In every area, he was rated a five which is the highest rating available. His supervisor, Captain Lawrence had some very glowing things to say about John. John, of course, is blowing it off saying it doesn't mean all that much.

He needed to get new ribbons and the new stripes for Master Sergeant so we went to a clothing store on base that sells all military clothing and accessories. He was in there so long I thought he had run into someone he knew. He didn't but it took so long because he had so many ribbons and other paraphernalia to get.

He tried to eat some mashed potatoes again tonight but could only get a few tablespoons down. Maybe it will be better tomorrow.

Tuesday, July 26, 2005

This morning John woke at about 8:00 AM. He was feeling quite clammy and sort of zoned out. He took a short walk came back and went to bed. I had showered and dressed then decided to get my nails done so I did not get back home until after noon. He was still in bed. When he did get up, he was better but still clammy. Took his temp and it was normal. He fed himself then we went to the clothing store to replace a damaged ribbon, dropped his uniform jacket off at "Alterations" to get the stripes sewn on, and then to the library and the post office. When we got back, he fed himself again and went back to bed. Just not a good day for him.

Last night I was doing the laundry and met a very nice couple, Gracie and Sidney. They live in Florida but only for three months out of the year. The rest of the time they travel in their RV. Sidney is retired Air Force and they have a son who is in the Army. He has three more years before he will retire so he knows he will have to spend another year in Iraq. He just came back from there after a one-year tour. They were telling me they had another son who passed away at age 31 from complications from Sickle Cell. They both said, that although it is difficult for them to say, their son is much better off now. He was in such severe pain toward the end, he just shook. The doctors said he would either die of heart failure because of the drugs or because they could no longer get blood for his transfusions. As it turned out it was the drugs that weakened his heart.

While this couple travel, they try to stay on military bases and they go and do work for their church, the Church of Christ. They did some work in Bowling Green, KY, at a youth home. They are finished for the summer and are on their way to California. All the work they do, they do for free. If building materials are required the church purchases them but the folks who do the work do it without compensation. They will do more work in the fall but then head back to FL for the winter months.

While I was home, I found out that United Dairy Farmers has stopped making Homemade Brand Vanilla Fudge Ice Cream. That is my mother's favorite ice cream as well as mine. I called the corporate office and found out they really can do nothing. I wrote a letter as did a friend of mine. Also, Roxanne is going to every Kroger she can find and filling out a request for that flavor and that brand.

Well, in the mail last week, I received a reply along with a coupon, but confirmation that they have in fact decided to no longer manufacture that flavor. Of course, they thanked me for my inquiry. Since no one could find that flavor anymore we all have been on the lookout for other brands with that flavor. I did find here in San Antonio, that Breyer's makes a vanilla fudge flavor. It is not nearly as good as UDF but you take what you can get. Of course, I will be following up with UDF telling them just that. Thanks, but we are changing to Breyer's.

John just woke up and it is 4:25 PM. He said he is now feeling so much better. He decided to put the last ribbon on the ribbon rack and one of the pins broke that holds the whole rack in place on his jacket. Now he has to go and buy another ribbon rack, remove seven rows of ribbons (which took about an hour and a half to put on) and start all over again. Nothing is easy for him.

The other day John put on a pair of jeans shorts and came out of his bedroom showing me how big they were. I knew he had lost some weight and had lost most of his gut but I didn't think it was that much. He let go of the shorts and they nearly fell off of his hips. He kept saying he didn't remember having a pair of shorts that big. Turns out he didn't. They were a pair of his dad's shorts that Ray had left here. We were cracking up at him trying to keep these size 40 shorts on his size 36 frame.

Wednesday, July 27, 2005

Today was yet another not-so-good day for John. He got up this morning at around 8:00 and said he felt kind of shaky. He is still having on again off again trouble with constipation. I had scheduled a bridge game and he insisted that I not cancel so when I left, he went back to bed. When I came back home, he had showered and dressed but was still feeling puny.

He says his throat is feeling better but he is still feeling as though he is being choked. He is getting really tired of the Boost but cannot get enough calories down without irritating his throat so Boost it is. His ears are still not as clear as they could be or as clear as he hoped they would be by now. Don't know what that problem is. Tonight, when he was getting ready for bed, he was saying how he was going to be so very glad when he didn't have to take any medications anymore. It is almost harder to see him with this much discomfort than it was to see him going through the radiation. And I am concerned about how he is going to feel next week and the week after because he gets his second of three rounds of chemo next week.

We went to the library and to get the mail and came right back to the trailer. While at the library, he had to make a potty stop and when he finished, he felt better again. Shortly after we got back here it started to get cloudy and windy. I didn't want a repeat of last week so John went out and rolled up the awning. Almost as soon as he finished it started to rain. We had quite a nice rainstorm, with thunder and some lightning. John says he cannot feel the trailer rock when the wind blows but I sure do. Not a good feeling either.

Thursday, July 28, 2005

Today started out to be a busy one for John. He had first to go to the Patient Squadron to see if his amended orders had arrived. Of course not. Then he had to get his labs done. Next, we were off to the TMO (Travel Management Office) to find out what he had to do to claim the expenses for moving the trailer. As he thought, he has to take his truck to someplace that weighs large vehicles and get it weighed empty. (The trailer does not count because it is a recreational vehicle and they won't pay for hauling it, other than some of the gas it took to get here.) Then he has to bring the truck back here to the base, fill it with the things he brought with him and take it back to the weigh "station" and get it weighed again. There is a lot of paperwork that needs to be filled out as well. I don't relish the idea of unloading this trailer and then reloading it again, but perhaps he will think of something different to do. In the meantime, he got a notice from Moody AFB in Georgia that the things he has in storage there need to come out or he needs to apply for a 90-day extension. If he does not have orders to return to Moody before those 90 days are up, I don't know what he is going to do.

I guess I am subconsciously revolting. The other day I was unloading the dirty clothes from the hamper and the top of the hamper snapped off. Then today as I was entering the trailer from getting my hair done, one of the vertical blinds snapped off. Honestly, I am not doing these things on purpose. Poor John, if I stay here for very long, he will have days and days of repair work to do.

John got sick again tonight. There seems to be a pattern here. He feels pretty good in the morning until he takes his meds, then his stomach gets upset. Same thing in the evening. This time he tried to take some Tums to settle his stomach and wound up losing everything. He is sure getting tired of this cycle.

Love, Affection and Blessings

K

Friday, July 29, 2005

Today was no better than yesterday. John did not feel well this morning again and he did not take any medication except the morphine. He called the Patient Squadron and his amended orders were in, so off we went. While he went to pick them up, I went to the pharmacy to pick up his refills. He was finished before me and when he came to meet me, I suggested he go get fluids. He seemed to think that might help and went to get them.

As it was going to take him at least two hours I thought I would go do the shopping. After I picked him up, he had to go to the finance office to file his travel vouchers. That took about 45 minutes then it was the library then back to the trailer.

Even after the fluids he still was not feeling well. Don't know what is wrong. He is just plain lethargic. He tried to inject some of the broth from the chicken noodle soup, but he couldn't take but one syringe full and he was done. He fell asleep on the sofa for a couple of hours while I fixed some dinner for myself. Don't have any idea what he is going to want to do this weekend, but I suspect not much. Then next week it is chemo all over again.

Tonight, I watched an NBC special about the niece of a dear friend of mine. In it her father, Terry describes his family going back to his grandparents and his own problem with alcohol. Talk about inspiring! He is an accomplished, skilled writer who can give you a wonderful word picture of a very difficult time in a family's life. One of the most tender moments in the documentary was when David, Terry's son said that his sister apparently didn't have room in her heart for him. That made me cry.

Saturday, July 30, 2005

Today was pretty much a repeat of yesterday for John. We spent a great deal of time today trying to think of what would be the best way to combat his pain without making him sick. One thing he is trying today is to take less pain medication more often. He is also doing that by feeding himself through the tube, less, and more often.

He is considering loading himself up with Triple Mix to, as he says, numb the hell out of himself, then try eating some solid food. I think he is slightly afraid to do that. For about two days last week, he got to the point of not having to carry his spit cup with him. Well, since Thursday, he has been hacking, coughing and spitting all over again.

Also, just under his chin, there is fluid building up and we cannot figure that out. Don't know what that might be. It has now been one full week since the tubes were put into his ears and there has been no change in his hearing. Still feels as though he needs to clear his ears as happens when on an airplane. So, on Monday he will be contacting the ENT doctor as well as his chemo oncologist.

One night last week, we took a short walk around the campgrounds. Just in front of us is a grassy area with trees and beyond that is a gazebo. On our walk suddenly a fox showed up on the grassy area. I guess it was headed toward the golf course which is beyond the gazebo. Didn't know they had wild animals on the base, but then why not? They have almost everything else.

Sunday, July 31, 2005

John seemed to be feeling somewhat better today. At least he was ok to go to church. After church, we had to come back here and get the propane gas tanks. Last night just before we were headed to bed, John noticed the light panel had a red light on it. He said we were out of gas in one of the tanks so he went out to change tanks. Well, guess what! He had no gas left in the second tank either! Ok since I know nothing about propane tanks, I am wondering how I am going to shower and wash my hair this morning. He assured me there would still be hot water. Non-believer that I am, I doubted it.

Of course, he was right, but when I was finished, there was no hot water for him! I asked if he didn't realize he was out of gas in both tanks. He said he thought he had SOME gas in both tanks when they left Valdosta. (They being Ray and John.) John said he was going to get the tanks filled there where he knew for sure they sold it, but Ray talked him out of it. Of course, Ray denies that. And naturally, it was a Saturday night and nothing was open and we didn't think anything would be open today. We did get lucky and found a U-Haul place that sold propane near here.

When we got back, he took in some Boost and I had lunch. Then I did some editing on a form I made up for him to fill out every time he injects or eats something. We are trying to see if there is a pattern to how he is feeling when he injects either meds or nutrients.

Library was next then back to the trailer. We pretty much laid around all day. John said he decided he really needed to try to get something into his stomach through his mouth. He said he saw me eating some cake and really wanted to try some but knew he had better start with something softer. Mashed potatoes here we come again. This time he ate a couple of spoons full then ate some apple sauce. You could see him grimacing but we both know he has to get beyond this. We were talking the other day about what the doctor told him which was if he doesn't start to eat pretty soon, his throat muscles will atrophy and he will have an even harder time getting something down his throat.

I knew he was frightened because he said before that when he tries to eat it feels as though his airway is closing. That has got to be scary. By the same token, I think he is feeling like that because the muscles are not being used regularly. I don't want to be a nag so I just wait for him to tell me when he is ready. Tonight, he was ready.

You know when you see your child, or anyone for that matter, hurting as John was hurting the other night it is so very frustrating when you can do nothing to make it easier. Remember when they were little and all you had to do was kiss it to make it better? Sure do wish that would work now but unfortunately, it doesn't.

So far, the food he ate, really ate, tonight has not had any ill effects. He still is not ready to try the cake even though that is what started the desire to try to eat.

Later tonight I insisted we take a short walk around the campground. He didn't want to go but I stood my ground and he finally gave in. I told him he needed to stimulate his bowels and walking was one way to do that. Here came one of those looks again. He said he thought he was the patient. I said I didn't want to hear about it. We took the walk.

I guess I wrote too soon. John just said his stomach is upset and his teeth hurt. The last time he put anything into his stomach was at 6:30. It is now 9:50. More than two hours later. Suppose there is a connection? Or maybe it was the walk.

He just now said he needs to force himself to get something into his stomach. Trying to keep the calorie count up. He went for the Boost this time.

Monday, August 1, 2005

Today John feels better. I can tell because I am getting lip from him. He is only kidding but he would not be doing that if he felt bad. Today, it is official. He is now a Master Sergeant. I know he feels good about that.

The agenda today was pretty much nothing. He placed a call to the ENT and is waiting to be called back. He had to have a blood test today and an EKG. This is normal just before Chemo starts.

He ate some more tonight. Applesauce and cottage cheese. Beats a blank.

We took another walk today, actually this evening after it cooled off. He was resisting but went anyway then decided to walk even further than I had planned.

Wednesday, August 03, 2005

The hiccups are back!!!! He started chemo yesterday and was feeling pretty good all day. Ate a scrambled egg and applesauce. Took a walk, but a shorter one than the day before.

Today after his chemo treatment we were on our way to the library when Dona phoned. The results of the MEB are in and when can John come to her office? We did a U-turn and went.

The board's decision is as follows:

"Your medical condition prevents you from reasonably performing the duties of your office, grade, rank, or rating. Since the condition has not yet stabilized, the Informal Physical Evaluation Board finds you unfit and recommends temporary retirement with a disability rating of 100% IAW Department of Defense and Veterans Administration Schedule for Rating Disabilities guidelines. The Board recommends a re-evaluation in six months." The key word here is temporary.

So, from the high on Monday of sewing on his Master stripes to a low of being told you are going to leave. John knew this was coming. I had hoped they would come to realize this was a bad decision, but then what do I know? John won't say but personally, I feel as though I have been kicked in the gut.

Now then, according to Dona, being given a review in six months is rare. She said he can go live wherever he wants. Unfortunately, she doesn't seem to understand he cannot because of being in this clinical study. He will have to live near wherever there is another hospital in this study.

If he accepts this recommendation, his orders will be cut and he could be out in 40-45 days per Dona. That would put it after the chemo treatments stopped. But she is also the one who said the board would take four to six weeks. She also said he would be eligible for Social Security Disability Income. That would begin six months from the date he last flew which was on March 10. The amount is based on the number of years he worked, his rank and the number of dependents. The SSDI would be in addition to his retirement pay.

He has three days to decide whether or not to accept the recommendation. He has to give Dona his decision by the end of business on Monday. Weekends don't count. If he decides to appeal, he will be assigned an attorney who will advise him on how to proceed. Right now, John says he is going to appeal, which everyone else has told him to do as soon as they found out his case was going to the MEB. According to what we have read, this really is not a bad thing for John but it is definitely not what he wanted. There is one flaw in appealing, however, and that is the appeal could result in a reduction of whatever the board has recommended. The only thing they could reduce is the percentage of disability but then that might be a better thing because if he is less than 100% disabled, he could be coded a "C" which means a "place limitation" assignment. On second thought, they could also increase the review to 18 months from six months.

To have this come at this time is just terrible. I said this before and I'll say it again. This is when he is supposed to be concentrating on getting over this disease, not worrying about whether or not he can stay in the service. I really think this is unconscionable. I may just have to write a letter to the Secretary of Defense!

So now he has to go to an office here called TAP, Transition Assistance Program. There he will find out things such as how much his pay would be, where his pay will be coming from, (I don't know what bearing this would have on anything, but John says it is important to know) what other benefits would he be entitled to, would the time out be counted toward his retirement should the six-month review determine that he could return to duty, etc. Then he needs to contact the Social Security office to get a figure on what the Disability income would be. He also needs to find out from the doctors, where the other hospitals are located that are involved in this study. He wants to know if Valdosta is not near a hospital, would his transportation be paid to return here to Wilford Hall for all his follow-up treatments? All this by Monday evening.

Even after this terrible day, I was surprised to hear John say he wanted, of all things, a hot dog! He ate the whole thing as well as some applesauce and that piece of cake he wanted the other day. Good job! He is really working at eating more each day and things that are not as soft as mashed potatoes.

It is funny sort of if you listen to John. When something such as this debacle comes up, his standard response is something like "I ain't worried about it." Can't stand it when he says "ain't." The other thing he says when asked how he is feeling is "Not too bad, all things considered." Says that even when he is really hurting.

Tonight, he said the walks really do not make him feel better, but he will go anyway. I think just to keep me quiet.

Thursday, August 04, 2005

Today, after his fluid intake at the hospital, he had an appointment with audiology to get his hearing tested. The test showed there has been a change in his hearing and according to the doctor it is from the Cisplatin he is getting. Hopefully, once he is finished with the Cisplatin the hearing will correct itself. It may not, however, get to a full correction.

We then went to see about letting Dr. Peterson know what the status of the MEB is currently but he was unavailable. We are to stop back tomorrow. I really don't know what he can or would be willing to do about this travesty.

We ran into Dr. Gallagher and John asked if she had the results of the CT scan he had done last week. She ran a copy of it and gave it to us. It reads, in part: ......" the previously enlarged retropharyngeal lymph nodes are less distinct and definitely smaller."

Something called the IMPRESSION states: "Significant reduction in the size of the left anterior chain cervical lymph nodes following radiation therapy. No new suspicious mass. Slight overall residual increased prominence in the parapharyngeal soft tissues on the left." I'm not sure I totally understand, but it sounds pretty good to me.

John had a check to deposit so we went off base to the bank and to the local grocery store. By the time we got back to the trailer he was wiped out, so he went to bed to take a nap.

Earlier today in between the fluids and the audiologist, he was hungry. I had some leftover spinach and that is what he wanted. He ate a pretty good portion. While at the grocery store, he said he would like to have a hamburger tonight. WOW! This is really progress.

Love, Affection and Blessings

K

Sunday, August 07, 2005

On Friday this round of chemo really caught up with John. He was so very tired that all he really wanted to do was sleep. He had eaten only a part of the hamburger the night before but he said his mouth was too sore to do much of anything else but take sips of Power Aide.

He was too tired to do anything about getting the information he thought he needed before deciding whether to appeal or not. We did speak with Maggie on Friday and she talked with Dr. Greene. She told us that Dr. Greene is the Surgeon General of the Hospital but even he can do nothing at this point. The only thing he can do is make sure the board understands that it would be in John's best interest to complete his treatment here.

I have prepared a letter to the Secretary of Defense and copied our Ohio Senators but have not sent it yet. John said we should wait until he is into the appeal process.

On Saturday, we spent almost all day at the hospital. He had to get fluids, get the chemo bag removed and get de-accessed. It takes about two hours to get the fluids but then the nurse wanted to run some labs to make sure he didn't need anything. As it turns out he needed magnesium. The doctor on call that day wanted him to get some by his port but since we had already been there three hours, and that process would take another two hours, the nurse said he could just use the pills.

By the time we left there it was 4:30 and I still had to go to the store. We got back to the trailer around 5:30. John took some more Boost and went to bed.

Today he got up but is still so tired, he is not going to church. This tiredness is not unusual. I am told that this is just one of the effects of chemo. His mouth is also sore again. Not as bad as it was with the radiation, but it is sore along with the back of his throat. So, he is back to not eating anything. And this will get worse the next time.

After church, I decided to go shopping. My mother's 90th birthday is coming up and I wanted to get her something. What do you get someone who maintains there is nothing they want or need? Well, I found this pillow that says" I'm in my own little world but that's ok. Everyone here knows me." I think I'll just get her a gift certificate for Kroger or something since she has been cooking up a storm for Ray while I'm gone.

What she doesn't know is John and I, provided he is feeling ok on Friday, are going to go home for her birthday. It is to be a surprise. My cousin, who had the heart transplant last February and his wife are going to surprise her as well. Ray is going to pick us up from the airport so we will surprise her on Friday. Then my cousin will be coming up from his daughter's home in Louisville on Saturday. Figured too much in one day would not be good.

John has slept most of the day. I didn't get home until around 1:45 and he had just gotten up. He stayed up for about 20 minutes then went back to bed. He got up again at about 3:30. I am just hoping and praying that he will improve by the end of the week and will try to eat something again.

Monday, August 08, 2005

John woke me up around 4:15 this morning saying he wanted to go to the emergency room. I knew it had to be bad if HE was asking to go to the emergency room. I flew out of bed and took him right over. Fortunately, at that hour there was no one waiting. He had been throwing up most of the night and had absolutely no sleep. The throwing up caused severe pain in his mouth and throat. The pain caused him to throw up more which caused more pain. A vicious cycle. They gave him some Zofran through his port along with some Morphine. They also gave him two bags of fluids. He quieted down but they kept an eye on him for several hours. His labs came back with a shortage of potassium so he had to get that put in through his peg and more morphine through his port. We finally arrived back at the trailer around 11:45.

After John had some Boost, I called Dona and asked for an extension. John was to let her know by the end of business today whether he wanted to appeal or not. I told her he had been sick and we had just gotten back from the emergency room. Of course, she had to call headquarters to see if they would approve the request. And they did. John now has until the end of business on Friday to let her know if he will appeal. If he does not let her know it automatically goes to the appeal process but without John's input.

John decided he would go onto a strict regimen regarding his intake of Boost and medications. He took four ounces of Boost every hour then 15 minutes later he took one teaspoon of morphine. He held to that for most of the afternoon but started to feel full so he moved to every 90 minutes for the Boost and 30 minutes later for the morphine. Then tonight at around 8:00 he had his anti-nausea medication. He wants to get up every two hours tonight to take some pain medication. He does not want to lose control of the pain again as he did last night. He was feeling a bit melancholy tonight because he thought he was going to feel so much better by now.

He decided he wanted to take a short walk tonight just to get out of the trailer for a while. We did and while it was still hot, there was a nice breeze blowing so when we got back, he suggested we sit outside and play a game of backgammon. He beat me, again!

John was saying tonight his unit in Iceland really had bad luck. In the past three years, one person was medically retired with a brain tumor, another had kidney stones, John being diagnosed with cancer and a fourth was just diagnosed with lung cancer. Something in Iceland do you think?

Tuesday, August 09, 2005

What a night we had. John wanted to get something into his stomach throughout the night so I set the alarm. Started at 12:30

then every two hours afterward. He alternated between Boost and Morphine. I am about bushed this morning.

He wanted to get fluids again today so after he had some Boost, I drove him over to the hospital. I decided not to stay at the hospital as I felt I would probably fall asleep and snoring in public is not one of my best features. I came back to the trailer and will probably take a nap.

Last night it rained along with thunder and lightning. Again, John put the awning up without asking. Guess he didn't want a repeat of two storms ago.

He called for me to come and pick him up and when I got there, he said the doctor wanted to see him so would I just park the car and come on in. Dr. Gallagher wanted to know what had happened over the weekend. After John told her, she suggested she give him a prescription for a suppository for the nausea. He just looked at her with this expression that said very clearly, not in this lifetime. She said I'll just give you the prescription to have on hand just in case. She also gave him a different prescription for a stronger Fentanyl and another for the mucositis.

By the time we finished with the doctor, got his prescriptions and got back here, it was 4:00 PM. Another day shot. We did manage another short walk.

Wednesday, August 10, 2005

John was feeling really well today, not good enough to eat, but good. Given that, I went to play bridge and he went to get fluids again. He did a lot of errands today as well along with some work here at the trailer. There was a leak in the bathroom sink which he fixed and for whatever reason, he felt the gas tanks outside needed to be washed. He also got some paperwork ready for both the leave to come to Cincinnati as well as a power of attorney for Ray so that he can accept the shipment of John's personal items coming to our house from Iceland. Truck gone, 600 pounds of personal items on their way!

One of the other things John did today was to buy himself a new uniform shirt. He needs to be dressed in his blues when he appears before the MEB (he has decided to appeal) so he felt he needed a new shirt since the two he has are from when he first joined the service. He also went to get a ribbon bar made for his shirt in addition to the one he already has for his jacket. He says if he has both, he won't ever have to remove the ones on his jacket. And I understand why. Those are a real pain in the you-know-what to get on. They have to be so many inches from the bottom of the jacket, so many inches from the lapel and so many inches from the sleeve seam. You should have seen us trying to get this all measured correctly with a paper tape measure.

Then after the ribbon bar is on, you have to measure the insignia for the "Maintenance Squadron" as well as his wings. On the other side is his name badge and that also has to be precise.

For whatever reason, tonight John has gotten the hiccups again. They have, in the past, only lasted three days. He had not had them since Saturday and suddenly here they are again.

I watched the special on Peter Jennings tonight. Thought it was very well done. When it was over, John wanted to take a walk. He said he thought it might do him some good. Since we had a real storm today, thunder, lightning, big, big black clouds and a pretty torrential rain, the weather really cooled off. It was a very pleasant walk.

One night last week when Ray called, he told me we have two hummingbirds. I am so excited about seeing them. We had gotten a feeder in the spring and I was so disappointed when none showed up. But they are there now. I just hope I get to see them before they start to migrate again this fall.

Thursday, August 11, 2005

This morning John drove himself to the hospital again to get his fluids. He said he was going to call me when he was finished as he wanted me to go with him to see Dona. He had some questions for her. Instead, he came back to the trailer and called her. She was able to answer the questions on the phone so that saved us a trip. He still needed to get his new ID card so we went there instead. We tried to go to the library but although the computers were working, they had no internet service. Yesterday the same thing happened but we thought it was because of the storm. No storm today however.

When we came back here, he was going to take a nap while I did the laundry. It was about 3:00 and I said this is the time to let me know if it was a go for tomorrow. He said we are going. The rest of the day was pretty routine including another short walk.

Our flight leaves here at 6:30 AM and they still had some seats left yesterday. As we fly stand-by it is sort of touch and go each time we go to the airport.

I am really looking forward to this trip even if it is short. We are going to celebrate four birthdays this time. My mother, Dale's mother, Marjorie and Benjamin (Roxanne's youngest.) Just as an aside, my mother said she would make the cake for Roxanne. So, the 90-year-old woman is making her own birthday cake. That, I am sure is definitely not the norm.

Friday, August 12, 2005

We made it! Up at 4:00 am, at the airport at 5:45 and on the plane at 6:25. We are now in Greater Loveland and delighted. My mother was sooo surprised! She doesn't know it but she is supposed to have another surprise tomorrow. Many things to do today so I am closing.

Love, Affection and Blessings

K

Monday, August, 15, 2005

Wow! What a weekend we had. Good and not so good. The good part you know was both John and I arrived from San Antonio on Friday without a hitch. My mother was so very surprised she was speechless. She and I both thought she was going to have a heart attack. Then on Saturday my cousin and his wife arrived and that was another surprise. We had a terrific time at Roxanne's and, of course, at her house the food was never-ending and wonderful.

On Thursday evening I didn't think we were going to be able to leave. John has a routine he has to do with his oral hygiene. There is a product called Prevident which he puts into his teeth guards and has to keep in his mouth for several minutes. Well, that night for whatever reason, probably the mucositis, the Prevident began to burn. He tried to keep this stuff in his mouth but in the end just could not. You could see the sores just popping out all over the inside of his mouth. After he had a bit of morphine they finally stopped burning and he was ok, but I was really worried for a while that we would not get there.

Before we left to come to Cincinnati, I received an email from our oldest granddaughter Stephanie, Tracy's daughter, asking if I thought I would have time to stop by and see her new pets. She has two turtles and a hermit crab. Well, I just couldn't wait!!! She wrote something about me holding these creatures and I wrote back I would leave holding the frogs to her Uncle John. Of course, they are not frogs, they are turtles and I just forgot but got another email to that effect. I sent her one that said sorry all I knew was that if you kissed one it would turn into a prince. No comment.

As she lives next door to Roxanne, my mother and I went to see the new pets. Stephanie took the turtles, Barney and Fred, from their tank and wanted me to hold them, but I graciously declined. My mother touched the shell. After Stephanie put them back into the tank, she used a hand cleaner before she pulled out the hermit crab, Jobo, I think is its name. My mother commented about needing to do that and I said it was because she didn't want to get any turtle wax on the crab. Grandma!!!!! These hermit crabs for those of you that are uneducated about this species are really ugly little things that hide inside shells. Any old shell will do. When Stephanie shook the shell, it started to crawl out of the shell. I'm out of here!

When we did get back to Roxanne's, Rachel, another granddaughter, daughter of Roxanne, said she had two hermit crabs and didn't I want to see them? Well, of course I did. Hers are larger than Stephanie's. And frankly, I don't remember if they had names or not but I am sure none of you will ever put me into the position of having to introduce you to them. Coming out of the shell, all three of them look like spiders and we all know how much I love creepy crawly things. Whatever happened to Gerbils, Hamsters, Cats or Dogs? Of course, there is a dog and a bird at one house and a cat at the other.

On Sunday after church Ray drove John and me to the airport. We were scheduled to leave on the 12:55 flight to San Antonio. We fly standby because Marjorie works for Comair. There was only one seat left on that flight and by priority, I should have taken it. I asked if I could transfer my priority to John and was told yes. So, he left and I said I would just get on the next one that left at 4:15.

The 4:15 flight was booked solid, as a matter of fact, overbooked so they slid me over to the 8:43 flight. At about 7:30 I checked at the gate and was told because of weather in New York, the flight was not even off the ground there and they were estimating it would leave around 11:00 PM. I was not about to have John come back and pick me up at 1:00 in the morning so I asked if they would put me on a flight for Monday, which she did. "Ray, come pick me up, please!"

At least the good thing is that John is back in San Antonio and able to keep his doctor's appointments. Also, he is well enough to drive. The bad thing is I cannot be there to hear what the doctor actually says. John's ears are not as good as they should be so sometimes he doesn't catch everything.

At about 2:00 this afternoon, looking at how many seats were still available on the 8:43 flight and how many were waiting to get a seat assignment, Ray said I should buy a ticket to make sure I was on the plane. I agreed.

John called to let me know that one of his doctor's appointments, scheduled for tomorrow, failed to get on the doctor's schedule. He has a second appointment with another doctor on the same day but they are 90 minutes apart so it should be ok.

While sitting at the kitchen table this morning, two hummingbirds came to the feeder. They are so very tiny. I had not realized how territorial they are. A third hummer came to feed and one of the original two dive-bombed the third chasing it away.

After I got to the airport tonight, I found a seat near the gate. There were many people there waiting for the flight before mine, going to Boston. That flight left at 7:15. About 20 minutes later with the area fairly clear, I look across the aisle and there sits a purse. I took it to the gate attendant and said I hoped the owner wasn't on the Boston flight. Turns out she was. The airport cannot call the plane to let them know anything. The only communication has to go through the tower. Later I was talking to the gate attendant saying how upset that woman must be knowing she left her purse and not being able to do anything about it 30,000 feet in the air. She let me know that the tower had been contacted by the pilot asking about the purse. The supervisor took the purse and they were going to put it on the next plane to Boston tonight. What a relief that must be for that traveler.

John met me at the airport tonight and we were back to the trailer by about 11:10. He got some very sad news today. One of the people in his squadron passed away. His name was Rod Mason. He has a wife and children. When we first arrived here, Rod had his mother send John some chocolate chip cookies. I just feel so bad about him thinking also of how nice his mother was to John. And how quick that was. He was diagnosed after John. Then another person died in Iceland. John doesn't know the details. This woman arrived there shortly before John left in March. So please say a prayer for both of the families of these individuals.

Tuesday, August 16, 2005

Today John met with the doctor who is replacing Dr. Peterson, Dr. Carlson. Turns out Dr. Carlson is from Ohio. He graduated from

Withrow and his family now lives near Madeira. He said he has a yearning for some Skyline. It just so happens we have a can so I guess we will drop it off tomorrow or Thursday.

His experience prior to coming here is with naso pharyngeal cancer at the University of Pittsburgh. He was stationed there prior to his assignment here. So even though it is a very rare cancer, he is still very familiar with it and the effects of it.

Anyway, he asked John all kinds of questions then he scoped him again. The scope goes up through his nostril then down his throat. The scope showed mucositis, a thick saliva, and something called the epiglottis being inflamed. The glottis is a part of the larynx and concerned with sound production. Lots of inflammation but no tumor. He told John it was imperative he swallow every day. I guess he is worried about the muscles needing to be retrained as was Dr. Peterson. He told John that the side effects may take twice as long as the treatment to begin to diminish.

We talked somewhat about the possibility of John staying in the military and he was not too hopeful. He did say that with John's type of cancer, if it does not show itself within two years, the possibility of it returning gets lower.

When we were talking with Maggie today, she said the prognosis won't be available for probably one to two years. I guess that does sort of go along with what Dr. Carlson said as well. All in all, John really liked Dr. Carlson. He is straightforward and to the point and does not try to sugar coat anything. Dr. Peterson was the same. Both were very willing to answer any questions we had.

He wants to see John again in two months which puts it into October. I am thinking that perhaps the appeal ought to center around the need to return to Lackland every three months for the next year and the travel would be a hardship if John were not still in the military. John has said on more than one occasion, there is a waiver for everything. Perhaps we can try for a waiver until at least the end of March.

Wednesday, August 17, 2005

Well, I am really a good one. I am supposed to be taking care of John's appointments. I had scheduled one for him for yesterday at 10:30 AM and of course did not put it on the calendar so we both forgot. It was with the TAP office (Transition Assistance Program) so it was not a major problem. John went over there today and rescheduled for next Wednesday. He found the name of someone who works for the Veterans Administration who knows what the benefits would be if John were to retire now on a medical or if he would retire at the end of March after reaching 20 years.

There is just such a change in John this week compared to early last week. He is sooo much better with the exception of being able to eat. He has been polishing his boots for the last three days. He cleaned the bathroom today while I was out playing bridge and has been faithful about increasing his intake of nourishment. He is now even trying yogurt through the tube and pudding that has been somewhat diluted with milk. He also told me he put Gogurt through the tube today.

John still has not gotten any of his mail from Iceland. We sent in two change of address cards plus his friend, Chris, sent one in right there in Iceland. They have very peculiar hours over there. They (the post office) are only open from 11:00 to 1:00 during the day, which means John has to call before 7:00 AM to reach them. It will probably get fixed about the time John is ready to leave here.

Thursday, August 18, 2005

We were on the go all day long today beginning at 7:30 AM. First, we went to the office in the hospital of the Texas Veterans Administration to see a woman who was recommended by the TAP office as someone who could answer John's questions regarding benefits on a Medical Retirement. She could not. But she said she would call someone and get back to John. We came back to the trailer where John took some Boost and a nap. At about 10:00 the woman called John and said he should go to the JAG office for his information. So, we headed to the Judge Advocate General's office. They said we should go to the Physical Evaluation Board. John declined because he does not want to stir the pot and these are the people who will be reviewing the appeal. The JAG office suggested we come back on Monday to meet with someone who was now retired but had experience in MEB cases. Now that appointment is set for Monday along with an appointment with Dr. Gallagher and Dr. Warren, the ENT.

Next, we went to the library. I cannot get to my address book. The technician came over and agreed to download the most recent Java update but even that did not help. I called Fuse and told them and they said thank you. We will get back with you within 24 hours. Yeah, right!

We then went over to the PJ's (the Para-rescue physical training area) to see Doug, a friend of John's who is going to take his truck to pick up John's new bike. For those who have any knowledge of the biker world, he bought a new Buell. They are to pick it up on Saturday.

Came back here to get something to eat. He injected and I ate. Then we took off for the insurance office in San Antonio so he could pay the insurance on the bike. He has been looking for about two days for the paperwork he printed off the internet with all the information on the bike but could not find it. I know it has to be here someplace but we cannot find it. The insurance agent had to call the dealer to get the VIN number and of course she was on hold for 20 minutes. She finally hung up, called again and this time got the number right away.

When we finished, John suggested we go to the movies. Well, I'll tell you after all the running today that is NOT what I wanted to do so I suggested we do that tomorrow. Can you tell he is feeling much better? This is the best he has felt since he had his first chemo treatment back in early July.

After making a trip to the BX we came back to the trailer and John wanted to actually try to eat something. I fixed him a scrambled egg, but it just didn't work. He gave up on food but he is still drinking something.

Love, Affection and Blessings

K

Saturday August 20, 2005

Friday, we ran almost all day. John wanted to get fluids so we were at the hospital at 8:00 AM. I dropped him off and went to do the laundry. It took until nearly 11:30 to finish both the washing and drying. I had just taken the basket out of the car when John phoned to say he was ready to get picked up. He had taken the can of Skyline in for Dr. Carlson and gave it to the receptionist to give to him. Of course, she forgot who it was for and gave it to Dr.

Peterson. He saw John later and thanked him for the chili. John said he was welcome but it really was not for him. Said he should keep it anyway and just tease Dr. Carlson with it. Best intentions gone awry.

We came back here and he got something into his stomach then we took off for the library. John found out that the airman who he thought committed suicide was actually murdered. I guess she was going to testify at someone's court martial but wound up dead before she could. They have a suspect but the investigation is not complete yet. How sad.

After a while, John decided to turn his mattress. This is not an easy task in his bedroom. I am trying to help him by standing on the bed and pulling on the mattress while he pushes. It was difficult but we made it. After it got turned, he decided it needed to be vacuumed. The vacuum he owns is worthless so off we went again to the BX and he bought a shop vac which he had been looking at the day before.

This morning he was up and dressed fairly early. As a matter of fact, he was up at 1:00, 5:00, 6:30, and finally for good about 8:00. He is also wearing jeans. It is 99 degrees here not including what the heat index is. I have been with him since April 11 and other than the days we were flying and the evening we went to the Air Force concert, John has been in shorts. He is also wearing boots, not sandals. Today was the day to pick up his bike. Now what would you think? My thought was he thinks he is going to be riding that bike even while he is on morphine. Not as long as I have a breath of air in me. He maintained he was only going to ride it here in the campgrounds. Uh huh. I said if he didn't want to be embarrassed by the ugly scene, I would make he would not even consider riding that bike anywhere but here in the campgrounds.

He was to pick up the bike at 10:00. We finally got out of here around 9:45. Now then, this is something John has been looking forward to for a year when he first ordered it. I know he knows exactly where we are going, right? Wrong! As a matter of fact, couldn't be more wrong!

He tells me we are going to take US 90 east to Interstate 37 North which we did. I asked him what the address was and he said he didn't know but you could see it from the highway. When we got to the Quarry we got off because he decided he should look it up and get an address. We had by now passed downtown which is where I thought it was but I also thought it was on Interstate 35 not 37. The reason I thought that is because that is where he told his friend Doug it was. Doug, remember, was taking his truck to pick the motorcycle up for John.

John came back out and said it was on Interstate 35 North. Mmmm. Ok now. Which way does he direct me? You guessed it, to Interstate 35 SOUTH. I'm just driving where he is telling me because I have never been there and he has so he should know what he is doing right?????

After we did yet one more turnaround, and it is now 10:45, way north of where we were and closer to the interstate that is near the base, we find the Harley-Davidson dealership. What we did not know is they were having a MOVING SALE today of all days. There are a gazillion people in there. Now if you are not a biker, which I am not, this is a people watcher's dream: executives, Iron Horsemen, tattoos, leather! Did I feel out of place? You Betcha! And now John is trying to tell me that is why he wore jeans. Right!

We finally tracked down Larry, the person who handles Military Sales and he looked very confused when John said he was here to pick up his Buell. Did you have an appointment? Yes, at 10:00 am.

Larry goes to check and comes back saying it is not ready!!!!!!! Not ready?????? Nope, not ready. No reason why it is not ready. Just not ready. Could we come back next week? To my utter amazement, John says, "Sure, I can't ride it anyway." John got on the phone to Doug to abort his trip. Hopefully, Doug will be available next Saturday. Did I say nothing is ever easy for John?

We spent some more time in there looking for a new leather jacket and a new helmet. By the time we left, it was nearly 12:30. We now have an appointment for next Saturday at 12:00 noon. We took a photo of John's disappointment when we got back.

When we got back to the trailer, he was on the phone with a friend who was going through a terrible time personally. He had called John for some advice. Don't ask John because he hates to give anyone advice. But he did talk to him for about 40 minutes. I had a sandwich and when he hung up he had some Boost.

Monday, August 22, 2005

Sunday was a fairly busy day again. After church, we stopped at Walgreens and as we were pulling into the parking lot, John noticed a new meat market. He said we were going to stop over there after we finished in Walgreens. Huh? He still cannot eat so I can't figure what's up.

What's up was there was a car in the parking lot that was for sale. A 71 Oldsmobile Cutlass convertible. One of his dream cars. He looked it all over and wrote down the phone number. It had a new engine and transmission. He called the owner and he said he had an offer of $8,000 but would be willing to consider another offer. John said he would have to think about it. Think about it?????

On the way back to the base, he decided he: 1. Really did not NEED another vehicle, he already has four; a truck, two motorcycles and a car; 2. Really could not afford another vehicle; and 3. Could only drive one vehicle at a time. Thank you very much!!! And not only was this the correct decision for John, but he tells me the person who made the offer had already gotten a loan for the car. Now that would have been a really dirty trick.

Yesterday afternoon John decided he needed to vacuum the whole trailer which he did while I did two weeks of ironing. Ironing in the trailer is a bit of a challenge as well as doing everything else in here. John took a photo of my "ironing board" and iron.

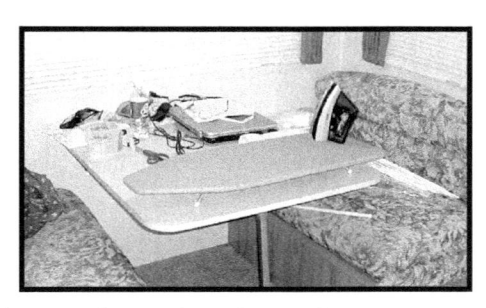

While John is vacuuming, he goes into one of the multitudes of storage places he has here and comes up with a box. "Guess what this is, Mom?" Can't. It is a pair of regulation shoes which he has had since boot camp. We are now going on twenty years remember? He must have worn them about four times because they still have the spit shine on them. He said something about spending four days shining his boots when all these needed was a touch up. He got out the shoe shine kit right away and gave those shoes a shine which only took a few minutes. He said he would finish the boots as well but not then.

Carole called and asked if we wanted to come over to play a little Euchre. We did and had a really good time considering we beat John and Arnold three out of five games. Carole made enchiladas for a "snack." Snack? It was a whole meal. Yumm.

This morning we are up and John is already polishing the boots. I went into the back room to finish dressing and I hear "Mom! Hand me the Fantastic please." What happened? "I screwed up." How?

You are not going to believe this because I wouldn't have if I had not seen it. It seems the polish started to dry out and was getting chunky. So, John decides to heat it up on the stove. Don't know how high the heat nor for how long, but it exploded and there was shoe polish all over the wall! It took him about 45 minutes to get it all cleaned off. When he finished, he was really pooped so he went to bed to take a nap. Oh, My! Just one more thing. But then I wouldn't have a lot to write about, would I?

Received a call from Dona this morning. John is to meet with the attorney on September 12 at 7:30 am. Then with the formal board two or three days later. She didn't have the name of the attorney. He will find that out when he gets there. This time the board is called the Formal Physical Evaluation Board or FPEB.

John had been told last week to return to the legal office today at about 12:45 to see Mr. Martin. Mr. Martin is an attorney who had been part of the FPEB process for about five years. The reason John wanted to see him was to find out what his benefits would be should he be medically retired. Given Mr. Martin's experience, he started asking John all kinds of questions. Then he gave him some very good advice as to how to prepare to meet with the attorney. That advice included contacting his commanding officer at Moody and asking if he would send a letter stating there is work for John to do at Moody. Letters from the doctors discussing how he has responded to the treatment, if he has been a cooperative patient, what his overall attitude has been during treatment, the cure rate, if he is capable of working once the treatment is over, the timing for recovery and for return to flying status would also be beneficial.

He also told him how to dress when he meets with the board, although John already knew that. He asked who was going to be John's attorney and when we said we didn't know, he said there were a lot of good attorneys there. I asked about the ethics of him calling one of them he particularly respected and asking them to take John's case. He said he would be more than happy to do that. He also seemed to think this could be dragged out long enough for John to reach his twenty years. I am not convinced of that.

Mr. Martin also did not have much to say of a positive nature about Dona. Even though he does not know her, he said she is working for the government and is really not interested in supporting the military person involved in this situation. Gee, I think we had already figured that out. The letters that John sent with the first package, according to Mr. Martin were probably not even read! That is exactly what I said to Dona when she called us with the results of the first board. Of course, she defended them and said they absolutely read each and every piece of paper. I doubted it then and am convinced now. Mr. Martin did say the next board is much more reasonable. In fact, they are looking for ways to keep you in the military if in fact that is what you want. Look, he said it is much better for the Air Force to keep you on active duty as long as you can work. If they TDRL you, (that means, Temporary Duty Retirement Leave) they get nothing for their money. If you are on active duty you are working for the money you get instead of just sitting around. Makes sense to me. I sure hope it makes sense to the people on the FPEB.

Later in the day John received an email from someone at Randolph Air Force Base. Are you ready? It states in part "…….issue orders sending member TDY to Lackland AFB, TX." TDY means temporary duty. It also said "IMPORTANT!!: Do not report to Wilford Hall Medical Center."

Do they even know where John is? I tend to doubt it. John said they probably think he is in Iceland.

He had an appointment this afternoon with Dr. Gallagher. She wanted to know how things were going. John told her his feet were tingling as though they were asleep. The same thing with the tips of his thumbs and his index fingers. She said that is the Cisplatin. If it hurt him, they could lower the dosage. He said no it didn't hurt, it was just annoying.

Next, he had an appointment with Dr. Warren, the ENT. After examining him the doctor said John has done phenomenally well. John told him that a couple of nights ago he was coughing and it was tinged with blood. That, said the doctor, was from the 5FU chemotherapy treatment. He has ordered yet another medication to help John swallow. He has also ordered another CT scan. Then he wants to see John right after the scan. He also said John's hearing had a very good chance of improving the longer he is off the chemo. Even with the tubes, John's hearing has not improved. The doctor did not seem to be concerned about it. After looking into his ears, his only comment was, "The tubes look good." Gee, that's good to know.

While waiting to see Dr. Gallagher, John ran into Dr. Carlson. He is the one who was supposed to get the Skyline chili. Well, he did get it after all. I guess Dr. Peterson gave it up without a struggle.

Tuesday, August 23, 2005

What a night John had. I just cannot figure this out. He has felt so good then last night he went to bed early and started coughing about 1:00 am. He was up at 1, again at 2 then again at 6:30. And after coughing up this phlegm for a while it began to show signs of blood. It was as though he really had to concentrate to get the muscles to relax to allow him to stop. It sounded as though he was choking. Between 2:00 and 6:30, I slept on the sofa because I was afraid he would choke in his bed and I would not hear him.

Looks as though this is going to be one of "those" days. The phone rang this morning at about 8:30. It was someone from the Reid Clinic which is across the highway on another part of the base. She had the audiology report and John needs to get that into his medical records. It just so happens he has his medical records with him for the interview he has tomorrow with the VA.

Then Ray called. The 600 pounds of personal items that are to be delivered to our house seem to be in limbo at this moment. He called the Destination Inbound at the Bluegrass office to give them directions and the woman he spoke with said she doesn't have a record of John's stuff. If we were in Clermont County she would, but since we are in Warren County that would come out of Wright Patterson Air Force Base. So yet one more glitch in the system to be taken care of. It just never ends.

After a few phone calls and a four-page fax we finally got SOME resolution to John's personal items. We are going to wait because Deborah, the person at the Destination Inbound at Bluegrass, said the normal shipping time to port is about six weeks. Then another two to three weeks before it gets to Kentucky plus another week or so to get to our house. Since the stuff was packed on August 2nd it will be a while before we hear anything. What was supposed to be a "nothing-to-do" day turned out to be a chasing from one place to another day.

John is feeling better now. Don't know what caused the problem but I sure hope it does not return.

John tried to phone his commander at Moody but wouldn't you know, he is on his way to Iraq. And the Chief is also TDY. While we were at the library, John emailed them. Just hope he hears something in time for the board.

Katrina hit the Louisiana coast today. Cannot believe the devastation. I have a nephew who lives near Keesler Air Force Base in Biloxi, Mississippi and a cousin who lives in Mandeville, Louisiana. We are a bit worried about them.

Thursday, August 25, 2005

Yesterday John had an appointment with the VA but he really didn't learn very much. They told him that they have a mass four-hour meeting every month and all his questions could probably be answered there.

Today, John wanted to get a shoulder and neck massage. He said it really did help release the tension and he is considering a longer and bigger area massage next time.

Also, John called Mr. Martin from the legal office this morning for some advice. A friend of John's suggested he contact the Disabled American Veterans because they very often represent patients before the FPEB. John wanted to find out if Mr. Martin thought that would be a good idea. He said it was entirely up to John but normally they represent Army personnel and not Air Force personnel. In addition, Mr. Martin told John that the person he wanted to represent John had in fact agreed to do so. And that is good news. John was told that when he meets with the attorney, he should be wearing his dress uniform. He is so very glad he has it all ready. He spent about an hour last night getting the nameplate, wings and maintenance insignia on his shirt. I never saw anything like this. But then I guess that is all part of the discipline of being in the military.

I had written a note to three of John's physicians explaining what Mr. Martin had suggested regarding the doctors writing letters to the FPEB talking about how John has responded to treatment; if he has been a cooperative patient, what his overall attitude has been during treatment, the cure rate, if he is capable of working once the treatment is over, the timing for recovery, and for return to flying status would also be beneficial. Dr. Gallagher phoned today saying she has written the letter and it will be waiting at the reception desk for us to pick up. She said John should read it and if there is anything he wants changed, to just let her know. She really is very nice.

Enough for this week. Next week John begins his third and last chemo treatment. Hooray! And Thank you God!

Love, Affection and Blessings

K

Saturday, August 27, 2005

Yesterday John had several errands to do. He was picking up Boost at the hospital, picking up dry cleaning, stopping by the post office, etc.

On Thursday John received this month's pay information online and discovered he had been paid nearly $2,000 too much. So yesterday one of the places he went was to the finance office to see if they could figure it out. They did. I guess they forgot to not pay him his flight pay and his Cost-of-Living Allowance which he was supposed to get while he was in Iceland. He has to write a check to them on Monday to get it repaid. He said he could just let them take out $50.00 per pay period but why draw that out? It's not his money and as long as he doesn't need it, he will pay it back right away.

This morning John was up and dressed by 7:30. He called Col. Pera, his commander at Moody who is now in Iraq. The colonel could not open his email so he didn't know what John needed. When John explained his situation, the response was "John, I would be happy to have you back in the squadron in Moody." He told him to call someone else at Moody and have him write the letter and send it to the Colonel for signature. The Colonel will then forward it to John. Things just keep looking better and better. I just pray he is not in for a huge disappointment.

John had to be at the Harley dealer at noon today to pick up his Buell. He was about jumping out of his skin he was so excited. I suggested he phone to make sure the bike was ready but he didn't want to do that. He said he would rather be there and if it is not ready, sic me on them. Well, no need as the bike was ready. It did take about two hours however just to get the paperwork done. And this was already paid for. He still had to pay the taxes, title and extra things he bought. As you know nothing goes smoothly for John. He gave the woman his credit card which is a debit card. It was declined. Now he knows there is no balance on this card as it is a debit card. He wound up using a different card, but now he has to take time on Monday to call and find out what the problem is. Not only is it inconvenient but it is embarrassing. The person who was taking care of getting it all in order was not the swiftest person but we finally got done. John could not wait to ride it so as it was in the front of the store and needed to get to the loading dock in the back, he rode it back there. I said that was the limit if he did not want an ugly scene. Doug arrived with his truck and a friend to help load it. As soon as we got it unloaded back here at the base he was on and riding once around the campgrounds. I know he was not satisfied with that short ride but he also agrees this is not the best time to be riding a bike while on morphine.

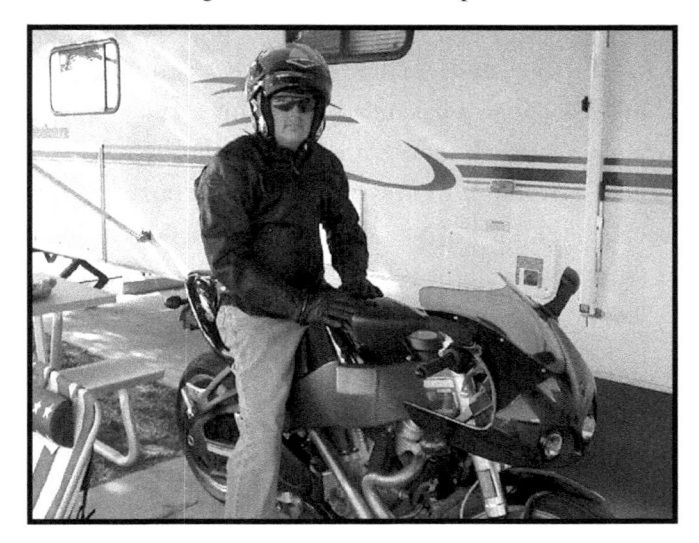

Doug's friend, Shawn, who helped with the bike, is in the Air Force as well. He was stationed in Guam, I think he said. He is a Parachute jumper or PJ as they are known here. On his last jump, he landed the wrong way and broke his neck. Where ever he was, and he couldn't say, it was misdiagnosed. I don't know what they thought was wrong but they didn't know it was broken.

About three weeks after the accident, he knew something was wrong, so he went to another doctor. (Can you imagine walking around for three weeks with a broken neck with no support?) They took ex-rays and there were two doctors in the room looking at them. They looked at the films, then at each other, then at Shawn. One of the doctors said "Don't move!" He went and got a collar and slapped it on him. They shipped him to Germany immediately and he was operated on there. He had a break in three of his vertebrae. He now has a plate fused to the vertebrae. He knows he will never be able to jump again because the same thing could happen again and he would be more of a hindrance to his team if he hurts himself when trying to save someone else. He has no desire to do anything else. John says PJs are very passionate about what they do and if they cannot do it anymore, they really don't want to do anything else. Shawn has only been in for about seven years so he doesn't have as much to lose if he gets medically retired now as John would have to lose. I guess he has not yet started through the MEB process but knows it is coming. He said he will be looking to John for advice when it does start.

After they left, we took some photos of John on the bike. There is also one or two of me. One of them has me in John's new helmet. I don't know how he can keep that on his head. Not that it would fall off but it is so tight and it is so hot here I would be a mess after five minutes. This bike is anything but comfortable. There is no back rest. The handle bars are about two feet from where you sit, so when riding, you have to bend over at the waist to reach the handle bars and try to hold your head up to see where you are going with a 30-pound helmet on your head. Talk about needing a massage when you are finished. Oh yeah! And this is supposed to be fun? John said this bike is built for speed, not for comfort. Oh! Just what I needed to know. Speed where? "Wherever I want to and don't get caught" was the answer. Another piece of information I didn't have a need to know.

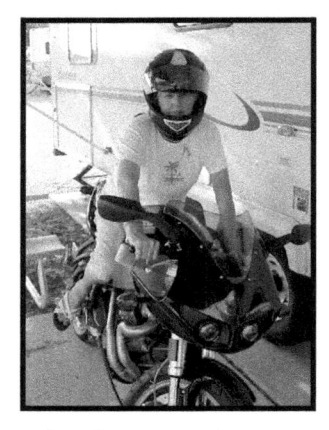

It was so very hot again today and I am talking around the 100° mark plus the humidity. When we got back here, John really needed fluids and he took about a whole bottle of gator-aid, through the tube, of course. He has been very diligent about keeping himself hydrated. Library and post office were next. There was a notice that a package was waiting for him but the window was closed by the time we got there. He will just have to wait until Monday. He hopes it is his mail from Iceland.

Tonight we played that new game Scene-it. He won again. He seems to like this game. It is fun and I enjoy it as well. The only problem is the DVD is supposed to automatically shuffle the questions each time you play but this time it didn't. We had mostly the same questions we had the other night.

Tuesday, August 30, 2005

Not much going on Sunday except Carole, Arnie, John and I played Euchre again only this time Arnie and John beat us two games to zero.

On Monday we were supposed to have just a quiet day with only a few errands to do. Those few errands took four hours. By the time we finished, it was around 3:00 and we were just then heading back to the trailer. John took a nap and I watched the devastation of the hurricane on the gulf coast. How utterly awful.

John called the credit card place when he got up and the answer as to why the card was declined was, they were having technical difficulties that day at that time. He should go back and try it again! He explained he had just used another card and said he would appreciate it if they wrote a letter of apology to the merchant for the inconvenience. "It is not our policy to write those kinds of letters." Evidently, they make too many errors of that type to make it economically feasible to be writing letters each time they screw up. Oh well, it worked out ok for John but just one more hassle to get straightened out.

Sometime a couple of days ago, while getting John's Boost ready, it got turned over. We thought it was all cleaned up but nooo. John opened the cabinet door under the sink and there found chocolate spilled on the shelves. We looked in the drawer under the sink and there was more chocolate. I had mentioned to John that the caulking around the sink needs to be re-done and now it is a necessity. The chocolate ran under the sink, into the drawer and down into the cabinet. That was a fairly good-sized clean-up job.

This morning John had to be at the hospital at 10:00 for the beginning of his last treatment. I started the laundry then drove him over to the hospital. Came back to the trailer and finished the ironing while watching the news again. This time there was a Coast Guard rescue helicopter plucking people off their rooftops. Quite a display. It is really unbelievable all the damage caused by the levees that did not hold to say nothing of the devastation caused by the hurricane itself.

I learned today that my cousin had to evacuate his home in Mandeville because it was underwater. He and his wife are ok, and that is good news.

Because of the extreme heat, we waited until after dark tonight to take our walk. We walked but just around the campground. One of the other campers came out and asked John if he was the one who had the Buell. They started talking and we were there for about 15 minutes. Turns out this guy retired from the AF in 2000 then he joined the Merchant Marines. Don't know when he left the MM but he and his wife are here looking over the base because she is joining the Air Force. She is supposed to be coming on board in December. Now why would you want to join the service when your husband just got out? He was talking about which career field she was getting into, something having to do with electronics. According to her husband, she doesn't want to be gone from her daughter for a long period of time. Just seems very strange to both John and me. He is going to take a motorcycle safety course so his wife can take the course. She wants to ride a moped. There is an advanced course starting next month. John seemed interested in knowing about that class since it has been a year since he has actually ridden a bike. He may take that course.

When John came back from the hospital tonight, he was saying that Keesler AFB in Biloxi, MS had closed. After Katrina, Keesler is about 90% gone. The hospital there is evacuating patients here to Wilford Hall. Because there are so many coming into this hospital, people who were scheduled to enter the hospital this week are being sent to Brooks Army Medical Center instead which is across town to the north.

The last two times John had chemo, Dr. Gallagher gave him Emend, which I believe I told you about before. This comes in a package of three pills. This time she gave him the same thing and five more capsules to take when the three are gone. Also, when he saw Dr. Warren two weeks ago, the doctor gave him something called Nystatin. This is a swish and swallow liquid which he is to take four times a day to help relieve the mucositis.

Another new medication is Promethazine AKA Phenergan. This is a new anti-nausea medication. He has so many different anti-nausea medications I don't know how he keeps up. I have kept a record of all of his medications. We are now on page four but that is in landscape format not portrait. There are 22 different medications. He is not taking all 22 at one time but they have been prescribed since he started this process back in April. Currently, he takes nine different types. Liquid Morphine and Fentanyl patches for pain; Zofran, Decadron, Phenergan and Emend for nausea; Nystatin and Gelclair for the mucositis; and Magnesium because he is low on magnesium. Of course, you can add Senokot S for constipation and if that does not work then he takes magnesium citrate which he gets at Walgreens. One bottle at a time but usually the first bottle works. If he doesn't turn into a druggie, it will be some kind of a miracle.

Thursday, September 01, 2005

The hiccups are back. They started out slow yesterday, but then last night they came back somewhat stronger. During the last round of chemo, John said he should eat slower and more often because that did not seem to upset his stomach as much as if he took in a full can of Boost at once. This time we forgot. So yesterday, he started feeling a bit nauseated. He did not get sick, thank goodness, but he did start taking in his nutrients slower. That seemed to help.

I was going to go shopping yesterday but by the time I was ready to go it should have been time for John to call me to pick him up. He is usually there about two-and one-half hours taking in fluids. I thought I would just wait and we could go together. This time it was four hours before he called. I could have done the shopping several times by that time. I decided to shop today because John was really tired by the time he finished yesterday so we just came back here and he fed Junior then on to the library and post office and back to the trailer.

We just sat most of the rest of the afternoon watching the devastation on the Gulf. I will not complain about living in this trailer again, I can tell you. Not after I have seen this. Words cannot describe what we are looking at.

This morning there were offers from people as far away as Boston opening up their homes for families. Some even offered bus fare to get them there. The people who see a TV crew are just enraged that no help is there but they have no way to know what is going on. It tears your heart out.

Then you see images of those people who are looting right in front of not only the cameras but in front of the police. Even the police were looting Wal*Mart. And some commentators were justifying this by saying they are taking the necessities. Would you tell me how guns, cameras and suitcases are necessities. Just makes me furious. Then there were reports of shots being fired at the rescue helicopters. Unbelievable!

There has been something I have been meaning to write about and keep forgetting. When Ray and I first arrived here in April there was a construction crew on a street across from where we were staying. They were digging up the ground and we had a hard time trying to figure out what they were doing. A couple of months later they started pouring concrete. It was too small to be the foundation for a building so we were still stumped. Then nothing happened for a long time. Suddenly there was activity again. And a brick bench was put in. About a month later the beginnings of a shelter-type roof object appeared. It turns out to be a bus stop. It has taken since about April 15. Today is September 1, and it is still not done! Our tax dollars at work!

John's hiccups tonight are really bad. He gets so very tired while on the chemo he decided to go to bed fairly early after falling asleep sitting at the table. I am sitting here listening to him hiccup in bed. I know first of all that it hurts like the devil to hiccup when his throat is so very sore and second it is just plain annoying because it keeps waking him up. If past experience is any indication, this should pass by Sunday at the latest.

Love, Affection and Blessings

K

Friday, September 02, 2005

John came back today from getting fluids and said the hospital is mobilizing to send people to New Orleans. Then we heard there will be more evacuees coming right here to the base. I guess this is in addition to the people coming to the hospital.

John had been doing fairly well this week except for being tired. Today is the worst he has felt all week. He feels very nauseated but so far has not really gotten sick. He is taking all the medications for nausea and the Phenergan which is to be taken as needed. He took one a couple of hours ago. Could be it is working but he just doesn't realize it because he feels so bad. Less than 24 hours to go and he is finished with the treatments. THANK YOU, GOD!

There is still going to be a long recovery time based on what the doctor has said but I know once this is behind him, he will be feeling so very much better. He has felt so good the last two weeks that I know he is feeling discouraged now but that will pass. We are just waiting patiently for him to be able to swallow regular food.

As I went out today, I passed the "Bus Stop in Progress." A crew of four people were working on the roof putting the tar paper on it. I was gone for about 90 minutes and when I returned, they were still there putting on the last of the paper. Now this has to be as big as six feet long and about three feet wide. Huge job, right? Cannot imagine how long it will take to complete the roofing.

Just as I was finishing dinner, (John couldn't eat anything) a huge storm came through. Lots of wind and rain. Lots and lots of rain. Of course, we didn't know it was coming so the awning was down. This time it stayed down and we just rocked and rolled only a little.

John just asked for some Tums thinking that may settle his stomach. In order for him to take them I have to put them into a plastic bag and crush them. Then put them into a glass to dissolve in water, then draw it up into a syringe which he then injects into "Junior." A few minutes later, he said he was feeling better. OK so we have all these high falutin' drugs and Tums is what make him feel a bit better. Go figure.

Sunday, September 04, 2005

Yesterday was a milestone for John. He had the LAST of his Chemo treatments. AMEN! Of course, he is not feeling really good because the chemo really drags him down. I know he is happy about it but he is still too sore to have that euphoric feeling that I kind of do. He is tired, his teeth, gums and throat hurt and he is being very cautious about how much he puts into his stomach at one time. He still needs to do as much water as possible so he does not dehydrate. Another good thing today is that John has not hiccupped once. I do believe they are now gone.

After church today, when we got back here, John took some fluids and went to bed. For want of something to do I cooked again. I have a taste for all the summer foods such as potato salad and tuna salad and marinated tomatoes. I know the tomatoes are not going to be as good as if I got the tomatoes from our garden, which we don't have this year, but they will have to do.

I'll tell you what, I am getting so annoyed at the stumbling blocks put in John's way, I could just spit. I think in the last email I told you about John needing a letter from the commanding officer at Moody saying there was a job for him to go to. This is for the FPEB which is next week. The commander is now deployed to Iraq so he asked John to ask someone else on the base to write the letter and he would sign it. John asked a Master Sergeant and he agreed. Then Katrina hit. John's old squadron at Moody was deployed on a two-hour notice to Mississippi. So far, they have done about 1,000 hoist rescues themselves. They had an NBC news crew with them for one of the missions.

Now the Master Sergeant was deployed with the rest of the squadron and did not bring his computer so he could not write the letter. He suggested John contact a major that was still at Moody and ask him to write the letter. John sent the email today and will call the major tomorrow. We are now getting down to crunch time for the letter as he needs it before the 12th.

And of course, John is really bummed out because he is not flying. He would love to be in the thick of this rescue mission in Louisiana. We heard the other day that there are 25,000 evacuees coming to San Antonio. Many of them will be at what used to be known as Kelly AFB, now known as Kelly USA. There was a DJ on the radio saying they need donations of any kind of clothing, toys, hygiene items, etc. We are going to go shopping and collect some of these things and drop them off at a collection point.

I so would like to be able to do more than just a donation, however, at this time it is impossible. I cannot imagine what the rescue workers are going through. Besides the people who have been affected by this tragedy, those volunteers are going to be needing psychiatric care I would think. I know I would probably get very depressed seeing all that up close and personal. I have a hard time even watching it on TV but it is like it was at 911. I was just glued and had to force myself away from the TV. I am sure many of you are just the same.

Monday, September 05, 2005 LABOR DAY

Today is not a good day for John. He feels bloated and is having a hard time forcing himself to take in fluids. I have been a nag all day making him inject something each 45 minutes or so but he finally went back to bed just to get me out of his face, I think.

I had said we were going shopping but actually we have done nothing all day. Tomorrow John has to go in and get his weekly labs done. He is supposed to go every Monday but with the holiday, tomorrow will have to do. We also have to go to the store for some more Senokot for John as well as those items to donate if he feels well enough.

Wednesday he has an appointment with a throat therapist to see what is wrong with his throat other than the soreness. Hopefully they will find something that can be fixed with relative ease.

Tuesday, September 06, 2005

John was still feeling punk this morning. Later I went to pick him up and there was a marked improvement. It really is strange how he can get dehydrated so quickly even while he is taking in liquids.

When he was at the hospital today, he told June, the nurse, that he had trouble sleeping the past few nights because of coughing up the drainage. Later I went to pick up the medications that his doctor ordered and there was a bottle of ten Ambien tablets for insomnia. All you have to do is say something is slightly wrong and here is a pill for it.

One of John's favorite programs is called "Overhaulin'" on the Learning Channel. They take an old car and completely overhaul it. I guess he gets tips on how to do some of the work on his truck from this show. Tonight's tip was: To remove road tar, use peanut butter! No lie.

Wednesday, September 07, 2005

This morning John went early to get his fluids as he has that appointment at 2:30. Yesterday he was at the hospital at 10:00 and was not ready to leave until 2:45. I came back to sort the laundry as I have not yet washed this week.

While I am sitting here typing the phone rang. It was the hospital calling to schedule an appointment for John that he already has for this afternoon. Oh my! Some of the redundancy blows my mind.

John's appointment this afternoon was with a Dr. Fairbanks. Turns out he knows Dr. Carlson. Anyway Dr. Fairbanks is in the Gastro Intestinal department. After talking with John, he decided to call Dr. Gallagher to see what exactly she wanted him to look for. He was afraid that trying to examine John's esophagus would cause John too much pain. And he was not convinced there was a problem beyond the back of John's throat. He even suggested John might be better served going to an ear, nose and throat specialist. Been there, done that.

In the end, after hearing John has tolerated a scope through his nose, he decided to do an Esophagogastroduodenoscopy aka (EGD).

How about that, sports fans? This is the description as written on the information page given to John:

"EGD is a test used to examine the upper gastrointestinal tract, including the esophagus, stomach, and the first portion of the duodenum." There is much more but this is sufficient. He is going to have this procedure tomorrow at 11:30 AM. Dr. Fairbanks did tell John they would be giving him a sedative. That is the good news because John's mouth and throat is so sore that he can barely open his mouth and absolutely cannot stick out his tongue. While sitting and waiting for the doctor to come in to the examining room, John said he was just a little nervous wondering what they were going to do to him this time.

Today was a really nice day. Did not get over 87° I don't think. Must be cooling off????? I was just asked about blood work and reminded that I have never discussed this in any of the emails. John does have blood work done each week. And just before the chemo treatments, he has an EKG. The blood work is done to make sure all his levels are correct and to detect any abnormalities. So far, the only thing they showed some time ago was that his potassium and magnesium were low.

Tonight, John took the triple mix to prepare his mouth for the Nystatin and you'd think he was being tortured, it hurt so much. He said this is the worst it has been. Unfortunately, this is the medication that will hopefully make it get better. His breath is also beginning to smell like a sewer again. This will go away in about a week but in the meantime ....

Thursday, September 08, 2005

John had to be at the hospital at 10:30 this morning. His appointment was really for 11:30 but they said they wanted him there 60 minutes prior. At 11:30 the doctor came out and said they were running about 30 minutes late. They finally took John back at 11:50. About 1:15 the doctor came out and told me that John was sedated but they could not get the probe down his throat because the opening was too small and the probe too big. He had sent up to pediatrics for a neonatal probe.

When it was over, the doctor came out again this time around 2:15 and told me that his throat is constricted, there is swelling and inflammation. It extends 14 cm and edema is present. Erosions were present. On the form he wrote erythematous mucosa.

In other words, the difficulty or pain in swallowing is from the mucositis, inflammation, and the throat being constricted. This should ease over time but Dr. Fairbanks wants John to let him know next week if he feels better and is able to swallow anything. If not, he wants to bring John in and give him a general anesthesia and dilate his throat. Personally, I think that would be too painful for John but then what do I know. Maggie called when it was over and when we told her what Dr. Fairbanks wanted to do, she also recommended against it.

I think it will begin getting better in another week just as it has in the past. The difference this time is there is no additional chemo to take place. In the past, each time he had additional chemo, those symptoms returned significantly greater than they had previously. The good news after all of this is, there is absolutely no foreign blockage which, in the back of my mind I felt was possible although not probable.

Ray is coming back to San Antonio around the 19th of September. We will be able to celebrate our 49th wedding anniversary together. Also, friends of ours from England are arriving on the 20th as well.

Please pray for John that the FPEB which meets next week, turns the original decision around and John is able to stay in the Air Force.

Love, Affection and Blessings,

K

Saturday, September 10, 2005

Yesterday was an easy day for a change. After John got his fluids, we went to the store and bought some stuff to take to church with us as a donation for some of the evacuees located here in San Antonio. One of the women at church lives near Kelly USA and she is coordinating a lot of the donations. Her husband is in the Air Force and was deployed on Thursday to Iraq.

After we got back and went to the library, we did nothing except play some cribbage. We did take a short walk too. The library brought good news. Colonel Pera, the commanding officer at Moody electronically signed the letter and it was forwarded to John. In it he described a job that he had for John to do back at Moody. This is something John has done in the past as a part of his duties as a flight engineer although he will not be able to fly. But it is a real job, not a made up one so that is good news.

When John was originally going through the MEB I did not have a good feeling and turns out I was right. This time I don't have that same feeling. I could say I am more cautiously optimistic about his chances of being retained in the Air Force. Only time will tell. I hope by the time I send this next Friday, we will know for sure. John meets with the attorney Monday morning at 7:30 and with the board within one-two days after that.

John spoke with his cousin, my nephew, about his home in Ocean Springs, Mississippi near Keesler Air Force Base. His roof is damaged along with mold and water damage in the bedrooms. They have lost some memorabilia, photos, etc. He told John the base was under nine feet of water. The good thing is no one in his family was hurt. I know they will have a hard time but they will survive.

Monday, September 12, 2005 (AM)

Yesterday after church John wanted to see if there was anywhere on base that was showing all the football games. Of course, he wanted to see the Bengals but there was nothing available. We went to the library then came back to the trailer and while John watched the football game that was being shown, I did the laundry. Hooray! The Bengals won as did the New Orleans Saints. That had to be great for the spirits of those displaced persons.

John is still having trouble with "regularity" so he has been taking magnesium citrate. Well, things finally got moving last night. We took a walk thinking that would help, then I rubbed his back thinking that might help. Whichever it was he began feeling much better almost right away.

This morning we had to be over at the FPEB office at 7:30 to, we thought, meet with the attorney. WRONG! I thought there was something wrong when I counted ten people in the room and only one person had been called back by about 7:40. Then a Mr. Smiley came out and introduced himself. He is one of the administrators there. He began by talking about the military people being there on TDY (Temporary Duty) and getting oriented. Of course, John is not TDY as he was permanently assigned here back in July. He called out some names on a list he had and sure enough John's name was called. He then told everyone when their appointment was and with whom. John's appointment is for 10:30 this morning with Mr. Butler. He also scheduled John for an appointment with the VA representative, Joe Nelson at 2:00 this afternoon.

On our way out the door I heard Mr. Smiley say to someone else that Mr. Butler is the head of JAG here at Lackland. JAG being the Judge Advocate General. Mr. Butler is the one Mr. Martin recommended John see. I just could not believe that we had to get up and out so early to hear the appointment was going to be three hours later.

Most of the other people were in their fatigues not the dress blues that John wore so he felt a bit out of place, but said he was not going to change for the meeting later today. He just wants to make sure his uniform is correct. One problem we are going to have is this meeting is scheduled for the same time when John should be feeding Junior so getting this timed just right may be a bit tricky.

Monday, September 12, 2005 (PM)

We met with Mr. Rob Butler. He is the Chief, Disability Law, Formal Physical Evaluation Board. He liked the letters John brought in from Col. Pera and from the doctors. He asked John to contact Col. Pera and ask for an addendum to the letter stating he is fully aware that John is not currently deployable nor on flight status, but that he is willing to have John work for him even with those restrictions.

Mr. Butler wanted John to contact his physician and ask him to contact the Flight Surgeons at Brooke Army Medical Center to get their opinion on John's prospects and what the timing would be to return to flying status.

He also said that I should be speaking with the people at the hospital with whom John interfaced over these past few months to get a statement from them regarding his willingness to have the treatment, how cooperative he was, how determined he was, etc. He even said I could testify if I wanted or write a letter. I think I am fairly good at writing so that is what I might do.

He gave John a list of possible questions John needed to be prepared to answer. This list is 12 pages long.

Then he suggested, when John asked about his uniform that John do something about either the tie or the shirt. John bought this shirt new and the collar was so messed up even the cleaners could not get the wrinkles out of it. Actually, there is too much material for the collar so it puckers.

Mr. Butler put us into another room to review the medical records. We did not finish until about 12:30. We left and headed to the hospital so John could get his labs done. While there I spoke with Jan the head nurse in the hematology/oncology area and asked if she would be willing to write a note about her observations of John. She agreed. Put in a call to Maggie for the same thing. Left a message. Then came back to the trailer where John fed Junior and I had some lunch.

While John was feeding Junior, he removed his shirt so as to not get any errant drops of Boost on it. When he started dressing, I just was cracking up. He had left his pants on so he put on his shirt, then unzipped his pants to tuck in the shirt but hadn't buttoned the shirt. So, with his pants unzipped he is trying to button the shirt and not having much success. At the same time his pants begin to slip down off his hips. While I am laughing, he looks up and says "I'm sure this will make it into this week's email." You betcha!

Off again for a meeting with Joe Nelson from the Disabled American Veterans. He started telling John about the benefits and saying he would get this much pension plus what he would get from the VA. I asked if John would get all of this if he had not reached his 20 years. Mr. Nelson was surprised John had not reached 20 years and backtracked on the benefits. I guess he misread the documentation in front of him. He did say that 20 or not one of the benefits available to him is a cross training benefit. If John wants to return to school, the VA would not only pay the tuition, books, etc. but they would give him a living allowance of $750 per month for four years. The GI Bill only goes for three years and they do not give you a living allowance. Mr. Nelson said that John could work even at 100% disability and if he were to apply for a civil service job, he would have a five-point advantage over someone who was not retired military.

He had John fill out all the paperwork as though he were going to apply for disability through the VA, however, since John would be applying in Georgia if he is not retained in the Air Force, John took all the paperwork with him.

After that meeting, we headed to the library where John got the email off to Col. Pera. Then to the clothing store to buy a new shirt, tie and tie clasp. John really resisted getting the new shirt thinking the tie would make the difference. Stopped at the post office to pick up the mail and headed back to the trailer at 4:45.

I write all this to show you what just this one day has been like. Mr. Butler also said to John he needs to tell the board on Friday what he does all day. Well, this is pretty typical. He needs to show how active he has been, if he gets tired from the medication, from the cancer, etc. In other words, he wants John to be able to say he gets tired no more than a person with no cancer does.

I am getting really frustrated because in my opinion the question regarding what activities he has been taking part in since being here is the most important. He has been doing a lot all through his treatment and he keeps trying to make it short, sweet and to the point. Well, he can't. It is just too important.

He did tell us two more things. One was that the MEB's recommendation was automatic for cancer patients. He asked if we had been told that and of course, John's "advocate" did not tell us that. She in fact tried, in a not-so-subtle way, to discourage John from appealing.

The second thing was that this whole process should have been started before John started any treatment. That is why the MEB suggested a review in six months instead of the 12 to 18 months because John is already six months into this treatment. Normally, if the process is started before treatment, they want to give the patient at least a full year before they review the situation. Also, when they review after the six months, they bring him back on active duty to do that.

Wednesday, September 14, 2005

Yesterday we slept in a bit before getting up and out. John wanted to go to the patient library at the hospital to see if there was any important email from his commander. If not, he thought he would call him. Later he decided against calling.

When we came back here, we worked on the questions Mr. Butler gave John. We worked on them the rest of the day. We decided to type the questions and answers so John can practice what he wants to say in front of the board. In addition, Mr. Butler wanted answers so he could look them over and run through the testimony process with John on Thursday.

John had written a note to Dr. Carlson instead of Dr. Peterson regarding calling Brooke Army Medical Center. We found out yesterday that Dr. Peterson's mother's grandmother's home was damaged in the hurricane as well as a huge barn on the property. These buildings are in Mississippi. Dr. Peterson is leaving here at the end of the month as he stored a lot of stuff in his great-grandmother's barn. The roof was blown off the barn so he had to go back to rescue whatever he could.

Dr. Carlson called last evening and said he wanted to see John today to discuss John's request. We went to the hospital at around 10:00 and saw him almost right away. He is really terribly conservative. He is very reluctant to tell John there is even a remote possibility he will return to flying status. He said in his career, he has never seen anyone who has head or neck cancer return to flying. Not good news for John. But then there is always a first time for everything. He talked about the possibility of other toxins showing up because of the radiation or the chemo that won't be known for a while.

He did however agree to write a memo to the board in which he said there was no further weight loss, (John has gone from 213 to 181) improved swallowing and decreased mucositis. He followed with this statement: "In my opinion it is too soon to determine a time line for when he might be able to return to flying status. It may be possible to make a less tentative prediction in three months' time."

This afternoon we are supposed to be going to go over the questions and practice responses. Hopefully, John will want to practice just a little.

One of the things I neglected to write about earlier was my experience driving the TRUCK. I put that in capital letters because as far as I am concerned it is a monster TRUCK. John said after we came back from the three-week break that he thought I could turn in the car and drive his truck instead. I just gave him the "look" that he usually gives me when I say something he does not think makes sense.

My verbal response went along the lines of "You need this truck to haul your trailer back to GA. You won't have it if I drive it. It is too big for me to handle. I could never make a turn in that truck. I would never get it out of the gate much less back on base if I left in that truck."

While we were in Cincinnati if you recall, he worked on the truck for several days. You must also understand that while in GA John had to put a new battery in the truck. Since he has been here, he has had trouble starting the truck on occasion. He thinks it may be the alternator or the starter but has not felt well enough to do anything about it. There was one day when I had the car and he had to go somewhere so he used his truck. Wherever he went, when he was finished the truck would not start and had to have a jump. And I am supposed to drive this????

One day, a couple of weeks ago, he said he needed to drive the truck around for a few minutes. It was while he was taking the chemo and I didn't think he should so I volunteered. He said ok and handed me the keys. He thought I was going to do this on my own! I informed him he was going with me.

First you almost need a step stool to get into this monster. After I got in and tried to start it there was a sound as though the battery was sick and had the dry heaves. It finally turned over and I put it in drive and away we went. As I was pulling out of the parking slot, I heard John say something about the curb. When I questioned, he tried to say it was nothing. I persisted and he finally gave it up that he thought I was going to hit the curb. HA! I cleared it with room to spare. John had me drive around the base a bit before heading back to the campgrounds. I was very surprised at how relatively easy it was to handle. I was expecting to have a hard time with the turns as I didn't think it had power steering but I was wrong, again. At the camp site the trailer is backed in first then there is room in front of the trailer for the truck. The trick here is backing the truck in and getting it close to the hitch on the trailer without ramming the hitch into the exhaust pipe, thereby damaging the truck. John got out of the truck to guide me into the parking space. I was ready to stop and he kept motioning for me to keep coming. I did as I was told and it was perfect! And on the first try! I not only surprised myself, but I am sure I surprised John.

Thursday, September 15, 2005

This morning John wanted to get to the library early to check email because he is looking for an addendum from the commander saying he understands that John would not be worldwide deployable and that is ok with him. Unfortunately, it was not there. We stopped at the mailbox then came back here so he could feed Junior. I left and got my nails done. When I came back, he was in the process of getting dressed for the meeting with the attorney at 3:00. We went over the questions one more time. On the way to the attorney's office, we stopped once more at the library. I decided to wait in the car. I opened both of the front windows to enjoy the breeze and started to read something we had brought with us. All of a sudden there is stuff blowing around in the car. There were some gardeners working on the grounds of the library and one of them was using a blower. You guessed it. "Oh! I'm so sorry ma'am, I didn't see you sitting there. I'm sorry. I got in trouble for this once before." He left. I got out of the car to brush not only myself off but the passenger's seat. In the process, because I was slightly peeved, I brushed too hard, hit the seat belt holder and broke a nail which I just had done about one hour before. Oh well!!!!!

We arrived at the attorney's office and did not have to wait too long before he came out for us. Almost as soon as we sat down, he asked if John would object if he, Mr. Butler went in with a summary instead of having John testify. John just looked at him. Then Mr. Butler explained. There is new information, i.e., the commander's letter, the letter from the doctor saying he is improving, etc. Mr. Butler feels he can make the case without John having to testify. John asked what happens if they don't go for it that way and Mr. Butler told him he would then come out, because we would be waiting outside, and bring John and me in and John would have the opportunity to state his case. John agreed to let Mr. Butler do the summary.

He asked Mr. Butler if he had received three emails on John's behalf and he looked and said no. He then explained that he has had trouble with the phone lines the past several days because they were putting in a new phone system. Now John has to find out what happened to the letters.

In the event the board does not buy what the summary states and wants to see John, Mr. Butler went over what will happen. He will enter the room first and sit down. Then John is to enter and stand behind his chair and salute stating, "Master Sergeant John Buckler reporting." I am to enter just behind John, close the door and sit down against the wall between the two tables that are facing each other. I was then instructed to NOT look at either Mr. Butler or John. I am to look at the three board members or down. That will be hard I know because I tried it while Mr. Butler was speaking to John.

Then John is to be seated and he will be asked his name, rank, social security number, organization, base and state. Mr. Butler then explained the board will introduce themselves, a Major who is the personnel person, a doctor, and the president of the board. Mr. Butler explained he will challenge (I forgot how to spell the word he used) the president of the board as she sat on the original MEB that recommended 100% disability and retirement. He explained that the two doctors on that board are very conservative and one more so than the other. He feels that if you have cancer, you should go home, lay on the sofa and come back to be re-evaluated in 12 months. He said the president of the board was probably influenced by their opinions. He also said that John could object to her being on this board but he knows her to be fair and she will take the new information into consideration along with what the doctor and personnel person thinks.

At one point John said he was attached to the Patient Squadron but he did not know what the formal name was for it. Mr. Butler said it was probably in his folder and had to leave for a moment to get it. When he came back, he said, "The doctor had your folder and I think I have good news. The doctor is right now inclined to let you stay in the Air Force. He has looked at your file and with the new information is pretty convinced you should stay. And the Major is usually all for the person staying in. In fact, he says 'If he wants to work, let him work.'"

He went over a lot more about what might happen if John has to testify but I personally was sort of in a state of shock. I am thinking to myself, "This is the chief disability lawyer. He could not hold that position if he had shoddy ethics. And ethically, he should not be saying this to John unless he is confident of what he is saying."

I don't know for certain what is going to happen tomorrow but I believe all of you have been working extra hard for our John. And we thank you, thank you, thank you! As for me, about two nights ago I just said "Ok, I am not going to worry about this anymore.

God, I am putting this in your hands and I am sure you are going to do what is right for John." Now I have thought about it but I honestly can say I have not worried about it. When we got up to leave Mr. Butler told John to not worry about anything, to not practice his answers, and to have a good night's rest. Sounds pretty positive to me, how about you?

When we left there, we went back to the library. Still no letter so John phoned two of the three people. They had not gotten John's original email. They both said they would take care of it right away. I called the third person as soon as we got back here and left a message then John fed Junior again. He changed clothes and we left to get my nail repaired and to go to another motorcycle store so he could look for a summer-weight jacket. Unfortunately, the store was closed so we headed back towards the base. There was a clamp John had seen on one of the awnings here in the campground and he saw that it helps with holding the awnings down during the wind so we went looking for one. Finally found one at John's favorite (NOT) store Wal*Mart. He also bought an accessory for the shop vac and as soon as we returned, he was busy putting the clamps on the awning and used the new accessory on the shop vac. Me, I am writing this while he works.

Friday, September 16, 2005

YOU ALL DID IT!!!!! The nightmare is over. I'll write more later about what happened today but suffice to say John did not have to appear before the board. They <u>approved his request</u> to return to active duty just from the summary judgment the attorney requested. There are still some hanging threads to fold in but for the most part the hard part is over.

We can all relax a bit now except to make sure the cancer is gone and the Randolph AFB review board accepts the recommendation. That will take about two weeks.

Love, Affection and Blessings

K

Friday, September 16, 2005 (PM)

What an emotional day this has been. Started out by going to the hospital to get some Boost. Then back to the trailer to change, feed, practice the questions and leave again in time to go to the library to get the letters that were waiting for the board.

John was sooo very stressed out today and I guess I was as well because neither of us had slept very well last night. I went to bed and tossed for about an hour, gave it up and got up and turned on the TV. John had gone to bed and when he heard the TV he came out of his room. I finally went back to bed around 2:30 and he was up at 3:30 and 5:30. Finally did get up to stay around 8:30. After our showers we began the day described above.

I must say John did look nice in his dress blues. When we got to the office of the board we went in and sat down. We were there about 15 minutes early. Nearly at 1:00 on the nose the door opened and a young woman called us back. My thought was "Oh no, it's not Mr. Butler. They must want to see John." However, when we got back there, she showed us to her desk and said the attorney had presented the summary to the board and John had to sign some papers. He looked at me and I at him with this questioning look. There was another woman at a desk and I asked what does that mean? She said "The board gave him what he wanted." Just like that.

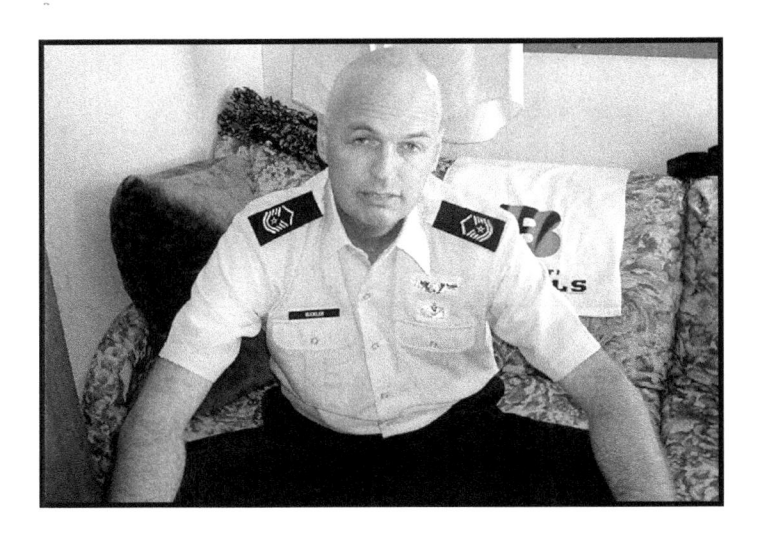

This is the statement as it appears on the recommended disposition.

"The member's contention was for Return to Duty. The Board notes the member has completed chemoradiation therapy with excellent response to treatment and not disease appreciated on physical exam during your 15 Aug 05 appointment. The Board also notes your strong command support and lengthy service. The Board opines the member's medical condition does not prevent him from reasonably performing the lighter duties of his office, grade, rank, or rating. The Formal Physical Evaluation Board finds him fit and recommends he be returned to duty."

We were not told a lot about the next step in the process but what we think we know so far is, John's file will be packaged up and sent to Randolph AFB. The review board there will review the recommendation along with the new information and either concur or send it up for review by the Secretary of the Air Force. I don't think it really goes to the Pentagon. If I remember correctly, we were told by the attorney that Col. Schwartz is the designated representative of the Secretary. Col. Schwartz was on the original MEB for John and was on this one. I really don't think she is going to reverse her own ruling even though she just did. And I don't believe the MEB is going to ask her to because of the new information. Maybe I am just too optimistic. But I still have a good feeling about it.

Anyway, John signed the paper, was given copies and we left. Just outside the door, John closed his eyes, head raised up and said "Thank you God." And I said "Amen." We could barely walk to the car. We drove over to the PJ Squadron to see Doug but he was on leave so we left and came back to the trailer. John fed Junior then went to bed. After all the stress of this week and today in particular, he just crashed. I don't blame him.

When he got up we went to the library to let the rest of the world know what happened today. When we got back here, we were going to get something to eat then head out so John could go to the motorcycle shop we couldn't get to last evening. We then just sat down and said we will go out tomorrow. We both were just exhausted. We did manage a walk but no more. I guess I felt almost as stressed as John but didn't realize it.

Saturday, September 17, 2005

This morning we got up and out early to get to the library as John had a couple of important emails to get out. Unfortunately, we both forgot until we got there that they don't open on Saturday or Sunday until noon. We were there just after 10:00.

The next stop on the agenda today was to go to the AAA office to get some tour books and maps for the upcoming trip. Ray and

I had decided to take our friends from England on a trip around some of the western states, including New Mexico, Arizona and Nevada. It is on the access road to one of the highways, 281. That is a road that you can see the signs for but don't have a clue how to get on until ooops, you passed it. So we did some detours and finally found the place.

Then we headed for another access road next to another highway for the cycle accessory shop. We decided to not go back the way we came because there was a major traffic jam going in that direction so John looked at the map and said turn here, turn there, etc. We were looking for a road called Wurzbach. We were up and down one road three times looking for Wurzbach. Finally gave up on that road and tried another. The second time around we see a sign that says, "Proposed Wurzbach Parkway." On the map there is no word Proposed. We spent around 20 minutes trying to find a way to our next stop.

Even with a map in the car we had trouble finding where we wanted to go. We were up and down Interstate 10 I cannot tell you how many times. Now you have to understand that John is, as I am sure I have said before, very laid back, just like his dad. About the third time around, he is beginning to get very frustrated. "Why can't I find that place. I saw it before so I should be able to see it now! This is really p-----g me off!" I said I was going to ask him a question that he was probably going to get angry with. "The last time we were looking for the Harley dealer you told me it was on Interstate 37 and it was on Interstate 35. Are we at the right Interstate?" YES! "Well, all that is at that corner is a shopping center. Is it in a shopping center?" YES! "Then why didn't you tell me that before?" Now I am beginning to get frustrated. We go back to the shopping center. John then says, "Now why didn't I see that before when we passed it?"

"Because you didn't tell me it was in a shopping center. If you had I would have pulled in here the first time we passed it. I was looking for motorcycles. Do you see any motorcycles here except for that one?" Would you say we have been together just a bit too much? I would and I know he would.

Ray and our grandson Bret, started out today for San Antonio. Having considerable experience traveling with Ray, I sort of know what he would like to do. He is one who wants to get from point A to point B with a minimum of stops including for sleep and/or meals. I told Marjorie she needed to tell Bret that Grandpa needed to drive for only eight hours and when they stopped they were to stop at a motel, get a room and sleep in the bed in the room. If left to his own devices, Ray would stop at a motel, sleep in the van, use the restroom in the motel lobby to freshen up then take off again. Bret was not inclined to challenge his grandfather on any of these points.

Tracy called this morning to let me know they left at around 9:30 AM. About 3:30 I phoned them and suggested they only had about two hours left to drive. Bret didn't want to pass on the message so I told Ray. He just laughed. At 5:30 I called again. Where are you?

In between Memphis and Little Rock.

You should have stopped an hour ago.

It's only 5:30 here.

Don't care what time it is, you have been driving for eight hours.

No, we haven't. We stopped for lunch, gas and potty breaks. That took about an hour.

Hey! The eight hours includes all kinds of stops. I don't care how many nor for how long.

They were pulling off the highway about that time and looking for a motel. They were supposed to call when they checked in. It is now 6:30 and no call. I'll have to call them and ask for the phone number and room number just to make sure they really stopped.

They finally called and are in Brinkley, AK about half way between Memphis and Little Rock. And at a motel. Down for the night.

Sunday, September 18, 2005

I called Ray after church about 12:30 and he was already on the bypass around Dallas. I guess they flew because Brinkley is nearly 400 miles from Dallas. As a matter of fact, they (Mario Andretti at the wheel) just pulled up and it is 5:10 PM. Anyway, they are here safe and sound.

This afternoon we had our very own sports bar minus the liquor here in the trailer. There were two games on TV so we had the set in the living area on then John brought the smaller TV in from his bedroom. Watched both games and were glad to hear the Bengals won again. We couldn't watch that game but we did get the scores.

Monday, September 19, 2005

We went out this morning and because Ray had driven for so long for the past two days and John had just had Morphine, I was elected to drive the truck. When we came back, I started to back into the parking space and Ray said he would get out and guide me back. John stayed in the truck and after I started back, John said I was too far to the right and I needed to line up the left fender with the edge of the trailer. Ok, so I pull forward and start to back up. Ray is in the rear of the truck motioning me to move to the right. Finally, I roll down the window and tell him I am only doing what John had directed me to do. Ray said if I kept going, I was going to ruin John's tires. OK. I'm done. I cannot take direction from two different people telling me to do two different things to accomplish the same end. I put the truck in park, got out and said "Someone else can park this thing."

I came into the trailer and sat down. Bret was still asleep. I turned on the TV and all of a sudden, WHUMP! The trailer shook. I jumped up and went to the door. John was directing Ray who was now behind the wheel. Ray said John kept motioning him to keep coming back. Well, he hit the trailer with the back end of the truck. Fortunately, he was centered and the exhaust pipe was saved. The license plate was a bit dented however.

Bret was still asleep. John opened the bedroom door and told him to get up. When he came out of the bedroom he asked why the trailer shook. (At least I did not hit the trailer when I backed in the first time.)

John had an appointment with Dr. Gallagher today. He had gained some weight and that is good. He told her about the FPEB recommending he be returned to active duty and she was glad for him. She did say however, she was not going to release him to go anywhere until he demonstrated he could eat by mouth. They would have to remove the peg and the port before he left also as she has no plans for any further treatment. She said, as did Dr. Carlson, that they wanted follow-up visits every three months for the first year. She is going to have him get an MRI within the next two weeks or so and has an appointment scheduled with him to go over the MRI on October 17th. He is seeing Dr. Carlson that day as well.

She also advised against doing anything about stretching his throat until at least a week or so from now. She said he should give the mucositis time to heal. He is really working at that with the Prevacid, the Gelclair and the Nystatin. She said the Nystatin was really a preventative against any fungal infection. I asked if an anti-inflammatory would be of any use and she said no because the swelling in his throat is from the mucositis. And there is a stricture which I believe is from the swelling. The bottom line is this is going to take time. I am not sure all of this is going to be accomplished by the time John would have to leave here for a report date at Moody of November 1st which is what he is asking for.

Wednesday, September 21, 2005

It is now about 4:15 AM. We are up waiting for Bret to get out of the shower so we can take him to the airport. Since he is flying standby, Marjorie thought this would be the flight he would have the best chance of getting on. It leaves at 6:30AM.

Yesterday I spent most of the day doing laundry and some shopping. I fixed a pasta dish for dinner and did some grocery shopping. Our friends, Maureen and Tom are coming in from England and Ray, John and Bret went to the trailer rental place to get a trailer for them. They spent the better part of the afternoon setting it up. Maureen and Tom arrived having had an uneventful flight from England.

Today I think Ray, John and Tom are going to work on John's truck. When they went to pick up the trailer the truck wouldn't start again and had to have it jumped. I think they are going to put in a new alternator to see if that helps. It is always something with this truck. It is about as trustworthy as a politician. You really want to believe what you hear but you know sooner or later the real truck will show its ugly head.

We are now back from the airport. It is 7:15 AM. Ray went back to bed. I am headed for an early morning nap. Bret got off all right. There were 40 seats available so there was no problem getting him on the flight. He couldn't believe it was going to take two and one half hours. I guess he forgot when he flew out here with his mother back in May.

Later this morning after breakfast Maureen and I went to the local AAA office and booked a trip to the Grand Canyon. It is a three day and two-night trip that takes a train and a bus. Stay at the hotel in Williams, NV. Sounds like a nice trip. Maureen and Tom have been here before and saw Florida and parts of the eastern and mid-western states.

When Maureen and I got back I started making salads for dinner for tonight. Then the phone started ringing. Roxanne first, then Roxanne again, then Marjorie. Everyone worried about Hurricane Rita. The plan currently is as follows, for those of you who might be wondering. Ray & I and Maureen & Tom will probably be leaving here on Saturday morning headed for El Paso. Should the weather turn nasty here, John's intentions are to close up the trailer, get on his bike and head to Carole and Arnold's home to ride it out. No one is going to be in a trailer during what might be 75 mile per hour winds. That is what they are predicting for San Antonio should the hurricane hit Corpus Christie instead of Galveston. At least that is what I think they are predicting.

Every hotel here in San Antonio is booked. The trailer park is nearly full, which I don't understand. I just spoke with Carole and she advised that we leave on Friday morning. She said if the storm hits Corpus Christie, San Antonio will be in for one heck of a storm and, because of all the creeks and rivers, major flooding. She said John should come to her house on Friday as well. She definitely does not want us to stay until Saturday because that day is to be the worst of the storm. I guess we might just take her at her word as she has lived in Texas all of her life.

John went to the Patient Squadron today to let the Sergeant, Karen Burrows, there know that the board recommended John return to active duty. She told him he must go to the patient advocate for the MEB, which in John's case is, you guessed it, Dona, and let her know that when she gets the paperwork from Randolph, they should fax it to Karen in the Patient Squadron. Once she gets the paperwork, she sends it to a place called Medical Standards. Don't ask, I don't know what that means. Once Medical Standards has it, John's orders can be cut to return him to Moody. John did find out that Dona is out on Convalescent Leave. I was very unkind and said she probably finally realized she didn't know how to do her job and it sent her over the edge. John found out from the MEB person who was there that he could go online and look up whether or not the code has been changed from 37 (medically disqualified) to a code C (location limited) also meaning he is not worldwide deployable. If he sees that the code has been changed, then he can notify the MEB to get the wheels in motion.

This afternoon the guys worked on putting on the new alternator. They quit in time to eat dinner and the discouraging word is the truck is still sounding as though it has the dry heaves when you start it, if in fact it starts at all. So tomorrow off they go again to get a new starter. Ray is determined to get the truck in running order before we leave on this trip.

Thursday, September 22, 2005

Happy Anniversary to Us! We had a different kind of anniversary day today as we sort of just passed each other all day long. We all slept in today. Poor Maureen and Tom have been having a really hard time getting their bodies used to this time zone. They both woke at 2:00 or 3:00 in the morning Wednesday and Thursday. They just sort of sit there looking at each other until they begin to feel tired again and go back and lay down.

This morning I got ready to get my hair done and was helping feed Junior when John said he thought he might be able to eat some cream soup. It was about 10:00. My appointment for my hair was at 11:00. Well, I scurried around and made a small pot of potato soup. Then I ran out of the door asking Ray to clean up my mess in the kitchen.

Ray was outside working on John's truck again. This time they decided to take the battery out, go to Sears, buy a Die Hard and see if that would fix it. He did agree to clean up after he finished removing the battery.

When I finished with my hair, I came back here to pick up Maureen and we were going to go to the BX. Unfortunately, she had decided to take a nap as had John. So when I arrived Ray and Tom went to the nearest Sears store. I had gotten some peaches and while everyone else was either sleeping or shopping I made a peach cobbler. By the time I got everything cleaned up, everyone was either up or back at the trailer. John decided he would try some soup. He was able to get two spoons-full down before it started to hurt. Later he injected two syringes full.

The guys placed the new battery in the truck but unfortunately it didn't correct the problem. They were trying to avoid replacing the starter. In order to do that, the truck has to go up on a hoist. This will not happen before we leave for this trip. And of course, Ray wants to get it done and John's response is as always "I ain't worried about it." Well, if he isn't going to worry about it, we shouldn't either. He has to haul the rented trailer back to the rental office on

Monday. He said the truck will start when it is cold so he will just not turn it off when he drops the trailer off. If it doesn't start, he will just get someone to give him a jump again. I am almost tempted to call Overhaulin' to see if they would do this kid a favor and fix his truck. Can you see us heading back to Georgia? Having to wait until the truck gets cold again before starting up after stopping for gas or having to jump it every time. A good thing I will be driving the van while Ray and John take turns driving the truck.

Some of them were hungry so ate some left-overs for lunch. We decided that we had better use up the food as John isn't eating and it will only go to waste. We will go out tomorrow night to celebrate our anniversary.

Hurricane Rita had been heading for Corpus Christie earlier so as I said we decided to leave here on Friday. Now it has changed course and is heading for the eastern coast of Texas and the western coast of Louisiana. We decided we would still be ok to leave on Friday morning. That is the plan as it stands right now.

My hairdresser was telling me that the shopping center where her shop is located has had a fairly heavy influx of people from New Orleans. They must be the ones who are staying on Kelly USA. Anyway, we are so insulated here we don't really know what is going on but she said that there were some who were very grateful for all the help everyone here is giving them. The downside is there are many who are acting as though they are owed something. They are harassing the shop owners if they don't have what the evacuees are looking for to the point that the San Antonio PD have been patrolling the center every day all day to try to stop this harassment. She also said that it didn't take long for the drug dealers from New Orleans to find out where to buy then sell drugs here. The one thing they did not count on is the Mexican Mafia. Evidently, they control all the drug dealers here and they didn't like the idea of someone else coming in here and not paying a percentage of the "take." She is afraid that someone is going to be killed before it is all over.

Love, Affection and Blessings

K

Friday, September 23, 2005

This morning after I sent the email John told me his code has been changed from a 37 to the code C we were looking for. Code C you will recall, means he is location limited because of medical reasons. This is wonderful news as it also means that the Randolph AF Base Board has concurred with the recommendation.

John now has to get a profile from his doctor describing what restrictions he is under. It then goes to the MEB who forwards it on to the person who cuts the orders. Dr. Gallagher will probably say he cannot leave until he can eat and he is restricted from flying for a certain period of time along with wanting to see him every three months.

Tuesday, October 11, 2005

We are now back in San Antonio!!! We had a great two-week trip traveling nearly 4,000 miles. I cannot believe we did that much driving but we did. Actually "we" did not do all that driving, Ray did. The whole trip. Let me tell you a little about this trip.

Ray started poking me at 7:30 AM while I was still in bed on the day we were to leave. I really don't like to be poked while still under the covers. After half an hour of poking, I finally gave up and got up. To say I was annoyed is a gross understatement. Ray: "Can I do anything to help you?" "Just stay out of my way!" I can be really ugly when I put my mind to it.

While I am in the shower I yell out: "If you really want to help me you can start by packing my clothes." Ray: "Where are they?" "On the sofa." "Where's the sofa?" "RAY!!!"

A few minutes later. Ray: "K, I really don't want to do this. You won't know where anything is." "JUST PACK!" A few minutes later. Ray: "You just want me to pack to have something else to get mad at me for." "No, all the clothes need to be ironed anyway. Just Pack!"

Later, John is lying down. K: "What's wrong?" "I'm just staying out of the line of fire. Staying out of the way till all the chaos settles down." "Chaos? What chaos?" We finally got on the road about one hour later than Ray wanted to leave.

We visited friends in Phoenix and took Tom and Maureen to Pinnacle Peak, a restaurant we used to go to while living in Phoenix. Went to the Grand Canyon and Las Vegas, with stops in between. At one point we were in a restaurant for breakfast and I said I was going to order biscuits and gravy. I wish you could have seen Maureen's face and Tom's as well. In England, biscuits are cookies.

At one hotel in Winslow, AZ On Route 66, which Tom was thrilled to be on, we were on the same floor but across the hall and down one room from each other. In the room directly across the hall from us we heard a dog barking and remarked that we hoped it was not going to be barking all night. Ray had told Maureen he wanted to be on the road around 9:00 AM. That morning, Ray looked at his watch and got the time wrong. He thought it was after nine when it was only a bit after eight. He called their room and asked how soon before they would be ready. They started racing to get ready and wanted to get some breakfast before they left. About 20 minutes later, I said I was going to go down to check out. I opened the door and here is Maureen and Tom standing by the door across the hall. There is a woman on the floor with a snake-like metal rod she is pushing under the door. I asked what was going on. Tom said, "We've been trying to get into our room for 20 minutes. The keys don't work." I said, "That's not your room. Your room is the next one up." There was stunned silence. They just looked at me, then each other, then the woman on the floor. "I don't believe it!" said Maureen. They both looked as though they wanted to fall into the nearest hole. There was an additional problem in that the woman on the floor couldn't get the snake- like thing out from under the door. It was stuck! She was going to have to call the occupants to warn them about the snake because they would probably trip over it and sue the hotel. And that was only part of our summer vacation!

John is feeling really good one day and not so good another. I don't know what is going on with him but perhaps this is normal for cancer patients who have completed their therapy.

He has been trying really hard to eat but without much success. He will eat two or three spoons-full of something or other but it gets stuck and he cannot get anymore down. He started out by eating some of the cream soup I made and went straight to Wendy's chili. I don't think he was ready for the chili. He has an appointment with the ENT doctor on Thursday as well as with the radiation oncologist. John has decided he is going to need his throat stretched so that appointment needs to be scheduled along with the removal of the port and the peg. I am sure the peg will not be coming out until he can eat regularly.

While we were gone, I phoned him one day and he said he had to attend a commander's call. What is that? "The commander has something to say to the squadron so we all have to be there." was the answer I got. After we returned to San Antonio, he showed us why he had to go to the commander's call. It was to receive the Air Medal Award. Actually, he has received one before so this was his First Oak Leaf Cluster. He was given this award for "Heroism While Participating in Aerial Flight." The document states:

THE UNITED STATES OF AMERICA

TO ALL WHO SHALL SEE THESE PRESENT, GREETINGS:

THIS IS TO CERTIFY THAT

THE PRESIDENT OF THE UNITED STATES OF AMERICA

AUTHORIZED BY EXECUTIVE ORDER, MAY 11, 1942

HAS AWARDED

THE AIR MEDAL

(FIRST OAK LEAF CLUSTER)

TO

TECHNICAL SERGEANT JOHN W. BUCKLER

FOR

HEROISM

WHILE PARTICIPATING IN AERIAL FLIGHT

"Technical Sergeant John W. Buckler distinguished himself by heroism while participating in aerial flight as HH60G Flight

Engineer, 59th Expeditionary Rescue Squadron 451st Air Expeditionary Group, 455th Air Expeditionary Wing, at Kandahar, Afghanistan, on 22 June 2003. On that date, Sergeant Buckler was launched on a mission to rescue two critically wounded Afghan Military Force soldiers, one with a gunshot wound to the leg and one with a severe spinal injury, located in a landing zone that was still receiving hostile fire over 200 nautical miles away. During aerial refueling, his precise power calculations ensured his severely power limited aircraft took on the maximum fuel possible guaranteeing enough fuel to reach the objective and return to the Kandahar Air Field hospital with minimum fuel reserves without the need for further aerial refueling. Enroute to the objective area, he recalculated critical power requirements ensuring his aircraft could perform the difficult brown-out landing with sufficient power. At the objective, Sergeant Buckler kept up an aggressive scan for ground threats in a persistently high-threat landing zone. Shortly after egress from the landing zone after his A-10 escort had to return to base for fuel considerations, Sergeant Buckler's aircraft received missile warning system indications of a surface to air missile launch. The crew successfully defeated the threat by maneuvering and dispensing countermeasures ensuring their safety and the safe return of the survivor. The professional skill and airmanship displayed by Sergeant Buckler reflect great credit upon himself and the United States Air Force."

We were all pretty impressed, Ray and I, and Maureen and Tom. John seems to think it is no big deal but I think it is more than that.

Also while we were gone the paperwork was all completed to be sent to Randolph so John's orders could be cut to return to Moody. He has not heard anything yet, but expects to sometime this week.

One of the really good things that happened while we were gone is that John used the last of the Fentanyl patches, and he has cut down on the Morphine considerably. He also has gone to the PJ's and worked out. He is planning on doing that at least three times a week.

I know he was glad to have some alone time and would like us to be on our way but he also knows we need to stay until all his procedures are over and he is back in Moody.

On Sunday night we had a terrific storm. The thunder and lightning were spectacular. It did scare Maureen and Tom, however. Guess they don't have that type of storm in England. Then it was overcast all day long on Monday. This morning it started to rain again and it is forecast for tomorrow as well. It has also cooled off considerably here since we left. It was in the high 90's when we left but is now in the low 80's. Wonderful! At night it really cools down. I have a very limited wardrobe for that kind of weather. Guess I'll just have to go back to Talbots. Whaddya think?

Thursday, October 13, 2005

This morning we met with Maggie and Dr. Carlson. There is good news and just a bit of not so good news. The not so good news is that John has lost about eight pounds since we left for our western tour. He has not been taking in as much nourishment as he should as well as not as many liquids. Ray and I both think he is in danger of becoming dehydrated again. I really got angry with him for not taking better care of himself. And what really makes me angry is he knows what he is supposed to do but just is not doing it. Enough of my soapbox.

The good news is the doctor scoped his nose again, which is very uncomfortable, and said there is no sign of a tumor. Everything he looked at, the vocal cords, the back of his throat as well as the naso pharynx appear normal. There is nothing suspicious. He then took his gloved hand and felt all around the inside of John's mouth and throat and said everything was good.

He did notice that John's mouth was very dry so he prescribed Pilocarpine otherwise known as Salagen which will help stimulate the salivary glands. The problem with this is, it is non-discriminatory in that any old gland may be affected. Some patients have even experienced diarrhea which would be entirely different for John than the constipation he had experienced. That, by the way, has gone away and he is back on the normal track again.

Maggie has scheduled John for several appointments in addition to the ones he had already scheduled. He sees the ENT physician this afternoon along with getting a chest X-ray. Then tomorrow he has an appointment with Audiology for a hearing test. On Monday he has an appointment with Dr. Gallagher and with Dr. Kennedy for a saliva test. The saliva test has to be done every three months for the clinical study. Then next Friday he is scheduled to see Dr. Fairbanks who will determine when he is going to stretch John's throat.

In the meantime, he needs to get the port removed, and once he is eating which won't be until after the stretching procedure, he has to have the peg removed. Maggie thinks John probably won't be out of here before the first or second week in November.

I am sure Ray will not want to stay that long. In fact, I know he will want to leave long before that. He has already said if John's report date is later than the 1st of November, he will go home then fly back when John is ready to leave.

Just returned from seeing Dr. Warren, the ENT doctor. John's appointment was for 1:00. They do things a bit strange here. John was considered a "walk-in" even though he had the appointment.

Seven Years Later

When we arrived, there were about six people waiting. All but John and two others were taken in and they finally called John around 1:40. A technician took us back and said they had a new system they had just installed and so everyone was learning and things were going to be slow. At around 1:50 a doctor showed up and examined John's ears and mouth. After looking at both ears he commented that John had a tube in his right ear. John told him there were tubes in both ears so he went back and looked in his left ear. Made me feel very comfortable. NOT!

He asked John when he had the most recent MRI and John said it was on the 1st of October. This doctor, Dr. McDermott, said because the computer in this room had locked itself up, (Give me a break!) he would have to go to another computer to look up the results. One hour later I am fuming. This is so outrageous having to wait for two hours before you see the doctor you came to see. Finally, I went into the hall and just stood with my arms folded and glared at anyone passing. The first person who got the full force of "Andi Anderson" asked if anyone had been in to see us yet. I said yes but it had been an hour and enough was enough. It was not a full minute later when Dr. Warren, Dr. McDermott and some other person who was not introduced entered the room. Apologies all around for the delay but Dr. Warren had been speaking with another physician who had a patient with the same condition as John. Evidently this other patient was not doing as well as John.

In Dr. Warren's words "John you have had a remarkable response to the treatment." He said that in the beginning he had told John he would probably need another neck surgery to make sure all the cancer was gone after John's treatment. However, because of the way the MRI looked, he wanted to have a PET scan done first. He seemed to think it would show nothing, but he just wanted to be sure. He said if there was even one cell left, he wanted it taken out. Doctor Warren said that the chances of the cancer showing up anywhere else but in John's neck was remote but he just didn't want to take the chance of a single cell being left behind. So now we think the PET scan will take place next Tuesday. We are still waiting to hear when the CT scan will be.

Dr. Warren also said he could do the dilation of John's neck if he was not pleased with Dr. Fairbanks. He said it would have to be done probably every three months for a while. Since John has to be back here every three months anyway, he will just have everything scheduled at one time. He does want this done the first time within the next few weeks so he can get back to work with nothing hanging over his head.

Love, Affection and Blessings

K

Friday, October 14, 2005

This morning, while I organized some paperwork and got it out of the way, John and Ray went to the gym to work out. They were back in what I thought was record time. Actually, they worked out for about 15 minutes which they both said was plenty.

John seems to have gotten the message regarding his intake of fluids. He is trying to do more and more.

He had his appointment with the audiologist this afternoon and since he was not actually seeing the doctor, I elected to stay in the trailer. While he was gone Ray and I defrosted the refrigerator and the little box on top of the refrigerator that we laughingly call the freezer. I have not had to do that for years. Don't want to do it again for many more years.

He said the audiologist told him there was minimal change in his hearing. Something less than .05 degrees. He also has his PET Scan scheduled for Thursday and the CT scan scheduled for the following Monday.

Monday, October 17, 2005

Today was a fairly busy day for John. He received a phone call saying his orders were ready, so he had to pick them up. Then he had an appointment for his saliva test, which will have to be done every three months. This afternoon he had his appointment with Dr. Gallagher. She seemed very pleased with his progress. She mostly asked questions which John answered. She also wants to see him every three months.

She did say he would have to have his port removed before he left and she put in an order for that while we were sitting there. She said he could leave the peg in until he was eating complete meals and not depending at all on the Boost through the peg. Then it could be removed in Valdosta. And speaking of eating, last night we had the pork chops cooked on the grill outside and John was able to eat a small portion along with some corn. It took him about an hour to eat that small amount, but he did manage to get it down. Tonight, we had angel hair pasta and he could eat that a lot easier than the chop.

His orders say he has to report no later than the 13th of November. That date happens to be on a Sunday. The previous Friday is Veterans Day so that means he will need to report no later than the 10th.

So far, his last appointment is scheduled with the ENT on November 2nd at 7:30 AM. This doctor also wants to see him every three months. Provided he can get the port removed and his throat dilated before then, and he gets all his out processing done before then, that means we can leave around 9:00 AM on that day. Hoooray! I think I can then be home around the 5th or 6th.

Luckily, Maggie will be scheduling all of John's appointments for the next year for every three months so John will only have to show up and not worry about all the scheduling. He will also have to have CT scans every three months for the first year. He said something about riding his bike here for his appointments. There are some things a mother just has no need to know and that is one of them. I think he was only trying to jerk my chain but I didn't bite this time.

Tuesday, October 18, 2005

This morning I woke to my phone ringing. It was the hospital calling to make John's appointment to have his port removed. It is now scheduled for Friday, October 28. One more down. Later in the day while we were out and about, John asked if we had ever eaten at a place called Rudy's in Albuquerque. We answered no and he said we were going to eat there tonight.

I wish you could have seen Ray's face. He was a bit stricken thinking John wanted him to drive to Albuquerque. And I sure didn't feel like riding that long. We might have made it in time for breakfast. As it turns out, it is a chain and John saw one on the side of the road on our way north. We found the place and turned in. We ate and headed back to the trailer. It was around 8:30.

Thursday, October 20, 2005

Today John had his PET scan. We thought it was going to take four hours and he was to have nothing to eat or drink for eight hours prior. His appointment was for 10:00 AM and he was back at the trailer by 12:30 PM. So much for four hours. We don't have any results yet but it is too soon. Hope to hear everything is normal next week.

An update on the "bus stop". I'll bet it didn't take this long to make the movie "Bus Stop." Passed by today and there is orange plastic netting all around the place. As I drove by, there were three people working. Well, let me qualify. There was one person with a garden hose, watering down the cement sidewalk which had been there for months and two other people standing around watching. There is still no sign of a sign stating this is a bus stop so I imagine that will take yet another month or so.

Tonight, John tried some salami, mashed potatoes, corn and applesauce. What a combination! He ate most of it. It takes him a long time to eat. I sure hope after his throat is dilated he will be able to eat steak and in a reasonable time. Today I was having peanut butter and bread (I also have a dietitian working with me, NOT!) and John was looking with lust at my food. I said I would not eat steak in front of him until he could eat it as well but I never promised to avoid eating anything else in front of him.

Friday, October 21, 2005

We met with Dr. Fairbanks today and he is going to try to schedule the dilation for Monday, if he can get the anesthesiologist on board for the same time. Hooray! Everything WAS working out as planned.

However, John informed me today he requested an out-processing date of November 5th not November 2nd. So that means we won't be getting home much before the 9th or 10th. I am not too happy with him at the moment but there is nothing I can do about it as the paperwork has already been signed by the commanding officer and cannot be changed.

He gave himself the extra time so as to make sure he had all his appointments done.

Love, Affection and Blessings

K

Monday, October 24, 2005

This has been an interesting weekend, to say the least. Late on Thursday afternoon, early Thursday evening, I felt as though I was getting a sore throat. I started taking Tylenol and continued on Friday and Saturday. By the afternoon on Friday, it felt like a full-blown cold which I had not had in quite a while.

On Saturday morning John decided he needed to get his truck weighed both full and empty. This has to do with the move back in June when he was transferred here. In order to get the maximum allowable weight, John wanted to load his truck with the heaviest things in the trailer. That would include books of course. All three of us were taking things from the back end of the trailer and bringing them to the door. At one point I picked up a small box of books and when I went to set it down, instead of doing it the right way, I bent over and POP!, went my back. I just crumbled. I immediately went for the Aleve and of course the ice pack. That did me in for the day.

Later in the afternoon, I was still in a lot of pain and John suggested I take some of his Morphine. I declined. He then suggested one of the Fentanyl patches. Since the Aleve was not working, I said ok. A few hours later, nothing. I am still in pain. John again suggested the Morphine and this time I said ok. I now have a whole new appreciation for how John must have felt while on this stuff. I have absolutely no idea how he functioned.

The good news today is that John is in the process, as I write, of getting his throat dilated. Dr. Fairbanks was able to get everything coordinated with the anesthesiologist for this morning right after John had his CT scan. I sure pray that it is only going to take once for this to work and he will be back to eating normally again. He has been eating but it is a very slow process for him. He can take a couple of very small bites, but then has to stop and try to clear what feels to him like a blockage in his throat. It takes him around two to three hours to eat something.

It is now 5:15 and Ray phoned a few minutes ago. John came down to recovery about 10 minutes earlier. Ray called about 1:30 to say they had just then taken him back to the operating room. As he was supposed to be there around 9:30 AM I don't understand the delay. And I guess I'll never know because I was not there. Ray told me that they had a lot of trouble getting an IV going for John to put him to sleep. They were going to do that first then put in a breathing tube so he would not suffocate while the procedure was taking place. Ray said they put two balloons in his throat area. Then there was another procedure the doctor did but Ray didn't get what it was. Another thing that took so long was, they took him to radiation to make sure there was no damage to the throat after the procedure. At least that is what I understood Ray to say. He also said they have scheduled John for this procedure a 2nd time on November 3rd. Dr. Fairbanks did say he would prefer to do this procedure every 10 days or so if in fact it doesn't work the first time. Please pray this will be the only time he has to have this done.

I have been invited to go on a weekend trip with 11 other people to Port Aransas. This group go every year and do nothing but eat, play bridge or poker and walk on the beach. They also go on a gambling boat one evening. I have accepted. It should give Ray and John some alone time and they can do some bonding.

Tuesday, October 25, 2005

John came home last night and although he didn't want to go to bed, he did nothing but sleep sitting up until it was time to go to bed.

John didn't get up until around 11:00 this morning and he has been very quiet all day. Just laid around again. He has not had anything to eat today except some ice cream. He tried to drink some orange juice but that hurt. The ice cream went down a bit easier. Hopefully he will be able to eat better tomorrow. He did inject some Boost. I know he is getting tired of the Boost. The next procedure he has done comes on Friday when they remove the port. Then it will probably be another two days of laying around because of the anesthetic.

Wednesday, October 26, 2005

John is feeling much better today. He ate a hot dog and some applesauce. He also ate some pork chop and dressing left over from the other night. He is still experiencing difficulty swallowing, but says the "shelf" he felt was in there is still there but a bit smaller. So that is a small, but nevertheless an improvement.

Friday, October 28, 2005

Yesterday I wanted to get out of here early to run to the mall but John said he would go with to get a neck and back massage. They have a kiosk set up in the mall for that. Before we left, he had to pick up the hard copy of his orders, go to the traffic management office to submit his voucher for the trip here then drop the orders off at another office. His orders weren't ready, he had trouble filing the voucher for the trip here, then there was another complication at the last office. Another example of bureaucracy at work.

Ray suggested we have lunch at the Cheesecake Factory. It was yummy but took forever. John was able to eat some Lentil soup.

John said that the blockage seems to be smaller and he is eating more of everything. Last night he had chicken and rice and did pretty well.

As we passed the "Bus Stop" we noticed the orange netting was down but now saw horses were up. This is taking longer to build than it did to build our house!

Today John had a 7:30 appointment to get the port removed. Ray went to the hospital with John. At about 9:30 Ray and John showed up. John was finished so soon. They did not put him to sleep, just gave him a local. He had a bowl of oatmeal and said he was feeling pretty good.

He said he ran into Maggie who wants to see him next Tuesday to give him the schedule of appointments that she has set up for him for next January.

John wanted some Tuna and noodle casserole for the weekend. While we were grocery shopping yesterday he decided he could probably eat that.

This afternoon John is going to complete the out-processing stuff you have to do when getting transferred out. He also wants to get his photo taken with a friend of his here, Doug to send to someone who wants a photo of John on his new motorcycle. I laughingly said he should "mistakenly" send the photo he took of me with his helmet on sitting on the Buell. He thought that might be pretty funny.

Love, Affection and Blessings

K

Friday, October 28, 2005

Tonight, while John was eating his dinner he started coughing and coughing. He coughed so hard he pulled a muscle in his back. I was in John's room watching TV when he came in asking where the Olbas was. I had no idea what he had done. When I found out he had already had Ray put the Olbas on. I said he should use an ice pack but John refused. It would make him too cold. So another chore tomorrow is Ray needs to take John back to the mall for another massage.

John said he wanted to wash the trailer and get it ready to move next week.

Tuesday, November 01, 2005

I left for the weekend of bridge and other fun stuff and returned today. We had a great time.

John had another massage on his back and his back is much better. He is eating crackers, potato chips and cookies in addition to regular food. I know this sounds good but you must understand when he eats these things it takes him a LONG time to sort of choke it down. He is still having the second dilation procedure done, however, the bad news is it is now scheduled for Friday instead of Thursday. That means we probably won't be leaving here until Sunday morning at the earliest. John said we might be able to leave on Saturday late afternoon, but we are just going to wait to see how he feels.

Wednesday, November 02, 2005

This morning John had a 7:30 appointment with Dr. Warren, the ENT. The PET scan results were NEGATIVE. Hooray! But then we already knew that. Dr. Warren scoped John again today and said there was still some irritation and mucositis but it was coming along very well. He said John's ear tubes would come out by themselves. He did say they will probably stay in for perhaps 18 months.

Dr. Warren wants to see John again in three months and said he would be having another PET scan in six months.

As it turns out there is a test, the spit, or saliva test which is required to be done three months after the radiation is complete and every three months thereafter. This is a requirement of the clinical study of which John is a part. It should have been done in September. Because John had such severe mucositis and the citric acid that he had to swallow would have burned his mouth too much, they scheduled it for October. It still didn't get done then, so Maggie has scheduled his return visit for December 12th. He will see the chemotherapy oncologist on that Monday and the radiation oncologist on Tuesday. They are going to try to get John scheduled on either the 12th or 13th with Dr. Warren. Sometime during that visit, he will have that spit test done.

We left Dr. Warren and went to Intervention Radiology to get the area the port had been in looked at to make sure all was well since it was removed. The following absolutely did NOT give me a warm fuzzy feeling. Dr. while looking and touching the area – "Have they started accessing the port yet?" In the first place, one can SEE where the port is when it is still in the body. In the second place, one can certainly FEEL the port when touching it. I am certainly glad he was not the doctor who implanted the port, nor the one who treated John for anything.

John was supposed to out-process today but as usual the bureaucratic nonsense overcame the common sense. "Sorry you cannot out-process until the day before you are leaving." But John is having that second dilation done that day. "Oh. Ok, well come back tomorrow." Now I ask you, 24 hours is going to make a huge difference to this base even though John is not working. When he came back and told me I spouted off and he reminded me he had been living with this kind of stuff for nearly 20 years. OK, I'll shut up.

Ray and John went to a place on base called Smokey Joes Barbeque for lunch today. I said I would pass. As I write this they are just now returning. If John was able to eat the barbeque that would be great. He just said he only had a baked potato because he was afraid to try the barbeque.

John had said he had a taste for sloppy joes. Haven't made that in years but I did. It took him about one hour to eat it.

Friday, November 04, 2005

Yesterday we had quite a discussion, Ray, John and I about where we were going to stay on our way back to Valdosta. Ray suggested we just pull into a rest area and use the trailer to sleep in. I am definitely not in favor of that. I just don't think it is safe. Then I suggested why don't we stay at a campground since I have become so accustomed to this abode. (I would much prefer a hotel but the parking might be a problem, getting the trailer in and out.)

Ray said there may be a problem with available space in a campground along Interstate 10 because of all the evacuees from the hurricanes. While they loaded the trailer onto the truck, no easy feat I might add, I went to the nearest AAA office and got campground books and maps from here to FL.

When I got back I started cleaning out the back end of the trailer where I have been storing all my stuff. I packed a lot but I still have all my clothes to pack. We want to clear it out so John can store what he usually stores there when traveling.

Today John was scheduled for the dilation procedure again. He had to be there at around 9:30. We arrived and checked in and were sent around the corner to a different waiting area. About 12:30 a nurse called John back. About five minutes later the doctor came out and saw me and asked where John was. I told him and he said they had been waiting for him all morning. I said we had checked in at Same Day surgery but they sent us here. He was not pleased and neither were the people in Same Day when they found out what happened. We could have been gone by the time they finally took him back.

The Doctor just came out and said all looked pretty well. He may have to do this again when John returns in December. He is still sleeping so I am going to send the email while he is in recovery.

This my friends, will be my last email from San Antonio. We will be heading east. I am not sure how long it will take for us to get to Valdosta nor how long we will stay there before heading home. I'll keep in touch and let you know.

Love, Affection and Blessings

K

January 24, 2006

Hi everyone:

I have had so many questions from people about John that I decided to send one more email to bring everyone up to speed.

First and foremost, John is doing very well. But I'll start at the beginning.

It took one whole day just to get out of Texas. We left Lackland on Sunday morning about 10:00 and finally pulled into a KOA just across the Louisiana border around 7:00 that night. On Monday we left about 9:30 in the morning and finally pulled into a campground at about 6:00 that night just west of Pensacola.

We had a relatively uneventful trip. I drove the van the whole way and John and Ray took turns driving the truck. At one point Ray asked if I wanted a break from driving as he would drive the van and I could ride in the truck. I graciously declined. I had ridden in and driven the truck while in San Antonio and did not relish the idea of bouncing along for several hours. I know Ray was trying to get out of the truck but I just couldn't do it. I figured I did the little apartment, I did the trailer, I did the 100 degree plus temperatures, I was definitely NOT doing the truck! So there! Selfish though that may be, that was what I stuck to.

We decided to go onto Interstate 12 around New Orleans instead of staying on Interstate 10. Then when we got to Mississippi, we stopped in Biloxi so John could go to Keesler AFB. He had some business to take care of there. The devastation we saw in that part of town was really unbelievable. You can watch TV all day long and not really get the full picture.

We arrived in or I should say near Valdosta, GA in a place called Grassy Pond on November 8th. Grassy Pond is the Moody Air Force Base campgrounds however, this one is not on the base as it was at Lackland. It is in a very quiet area with lots and lots of trees. There is a separate area that has cabins and, of course, the pond or small lake.

The next day we headed to the base to unload the motorcycle from the truck, go to the library and the housing office. Then we picked up John's children for dinner. At the housing office John was looking for houses for sale in the area. He had decided to buy a house rather than use base housing or rent a place which is like throwing money away. He needed a place big enough so his children would have a place to stay when they come to him every other weekend.

He wound up liking the very first house he saw and it was definitely within his price range. Ray and I stayed until Friday and left for Cincinnati on the 11th of November. We spent the night in a hotel just north of Atlanta as it had taken us two and one half hours to get through Atlanta. There had been a rain storm and the traffic was just unbelievable. We finally arrived back in Loveland on Saturday the 12th after seven months (essentially) in Texas.

I cannot express to you how great it was to be home again. But then we went right into the Thanksgiving and Christmas holidays and it was kind of a whirlwind. I sort of felt like a whirling dervish by the time January 2nd came and went.

In December John had to go back to San Antonio for his three-month check-up. He was pronounced fit except for his hearing. He has lost more hearing and they fitted him for hearing aids which he will get when he goes back in March. He was told they had radiated him through his inner ear. We did not know that while the radiation was going on. We don't know if any of his hearing will return and neither do the doctors. That will be known over time. He had another throat dilation and this time he said he noticed a definite improvement; much more than the first two times. He arrived back in Georgia in time to pick up his children and head north for Christmas.

They arrived here in Loveland on Monday the 19th. It was great to have them here for the holiday. They did a lot of running around, paint balling, skiing, etc. And they spent a lot of time with Marjorie and her children.

John and Ray and John's children spent the whole day on Friday loading the utility trailer John had left here in 2003 just before he went to Iceland, with all his stuff. And he had a lot of stuff. Among other things he had his Goldwing Motorcycle here along with a chest of drawers, a cedar chest, two lawn mowers and three huge boxes of household goods that were shipped here from Iceland. I really don't know how they got everything on the trailer and/or into the truck but they did.

John had to leave on Monday the 26th of December because his daughter, Gemma had to leave Valdosta on Tuesday the 27th for Pasadena. Her high school band, of which she is a part, was invited to play in the Rose Bowl Parade. She was really very excited about going. In the process of getting out of here John forgot all of his oral hygiene stuff which he needed asap, so we wound up overnighting it to him on Tuesday. Then the next day he called and said he had left all of his medical records here. No overnight this time. Just regular mail.

As soon as John got back to Valdosta, he closed on the house he had made an offer on. He took possession on the 2nd of January. He had told the owners that he would pay for their closing costs if they would have the house cleaned. The owner was getting out of the Air Force but had never lived in base housing. When you live in base housing and move you are expected to clean or have the house cleaned to "white glove" standards. Never having lived in base housing, these owners just did the usual cleaning and it was not what John had expected so he had a lot of work to do before he could move in.

He pulled his trailer up from Grassy Pond to the driveway and lived in it for a couple of weeks until he got it sort of where he wanted it.

In the meantime, his flight surgeon gave him a physical and said as soon as John gains some weight and gains some strength back, he should be fit to fly again. Is that great or what????? Regarding his hearing, he said at that time he, the flight surgeon, would take John out to the flight line and with the engines running, give John a hearing test. If his hearing is not too bad, he would apply for a waiver for John to be able to fly.

John told Ray he was going to take up the carpeting in the living room and the tile from the kitchen and bathroom as well as the tile from in front of the front door and replace it all with other tile and/or hardwood flooring. He also wants to paint. He did have his children paint their rooms. Gemma chose black with some kind of designs on the walls and Dean chose green and yellow, which are the hazardous waste colors. Oh well, to each his own.

John asked Ray if he would come down and help him with this work or Ray volunteered, I'm not sure which. Ray left here on Tuesday the 16th of January. He is working his buns off I am told. A few days before Ray went out there John had Dean and Trent, his youngest, to Dean's paint ball tournament. There is something called an air barrier. It is something the players can run into and not get hurt. One of these barriers was laying on the ground and some of the children who were not participants were playing on this barrier, Trent among them. One of the other children jumped on one end of the barrier and Trent was on the other end. It acted like a see-saw and Trent went flying up into the air and came down the wrong way and broke his arm. Little trouper that he is, he didn't complain too much even when they had to set it. He is doing well now.

Again before Ray left, John called one day and asked if I was coming down with Ray to help "organize" his kitchen. Ray quietly said "No, your mother is pretty busy." Let Ray have his turn in the barrel.

It seems they had a bit of excitement at the house in Valdosta last week. I mentioned John wanted to take up the tile in the house and replace it. There was tile at the front entrance which Ray took up. This tile had been glued down with some sort of substance which when dried, turns to cement or something very like cement. Ray worked trying to get this stuff up off the flooring but it wasn't an easy task even with a hammer and chisel. John then decided to use his sander to get it up. Now then, I don't think either one of them thought to open the door or a window. John is happily sanding away and creating so much dust that suddenly the smoke alarm goes off. This alarm is hooked up to an alarm company which John never activated. Suddenly a voice is yelling "There is a fire! Get out of the house. There is a fire! Get out of the house."

Ray is very laid back and does not get excited about anything. Well, John is the same way. I told you before, his favorite phrase is "I ain't worried about it." They did not tell me exactly what happened but I can just picture the two of them looking at each other, scratching their heads and asking "What is that?" They could not figure out what the code was to turn off this wonderful alarm and by the way I have never heard of an alarm with a recording which says "There is a fire! Get out of the house." Never the less, they both are going around the house looking for a button or switch to turn this off but could not find one. Finally on one of the alarm boxes there was a phone number which John called and they told him how to disconnect it. I don't know if they thought it was funny or not but I'll tell you I sure did.

Last week John had an in-flight hearing test. There are two parts to this test. The first is a word test. John is given a piece of paper with 100 groups of three words in a group. With his headphones on and the engines running, someone says a word to John. He is to pick out the word from one of these 100 groups of words. The second test is a phrase test where someone gives John a phrase and John is to repeat it back to whomever. There are 50 phrases given in this test.

In the first test, out of 100 words, John missed six and out of 50 phrases John missed one. I thought that was pretty good but John said it is not a pass or fail test. What they will do is compare it, mathematically with scores of others who have no hearing problem to determine if he can fly without the waiver. If he needs the waiver, they will apply for one but he won't know what is going to happen until the end of February or beginning of March.

Ray said John is still very tired when he gets home from work but now they have moved him to a different squadron and he has to go do exercise each morning at 7:00 AM. That may help him to not feel so tired at the end of the day.

John is also going TDY (temporary duty assignment) to Tucson on February 5th for a week. Ray at first thought he would come home then go back later. Yesterday he said he might be staying just to get it over with so he doesn't have to go back.

With Love, Affection and Blessings

K

That was the last email I sent.

EPILOGUE

After John was reassigned to Moody Air Force Base in 2005, he was assigned to Air Combat Command and was able stay in his career field. He became fully mission capable and obtained waivers to return to flying status from the Secretary of the Air Force and deploy two more times. He also obtained one more waiver to stay in the Air Force for one additional year. When he was fully mission capable, John's commander sent for a journalist to do a profile on John. It was published in the Air Force News along with a couple of photos.

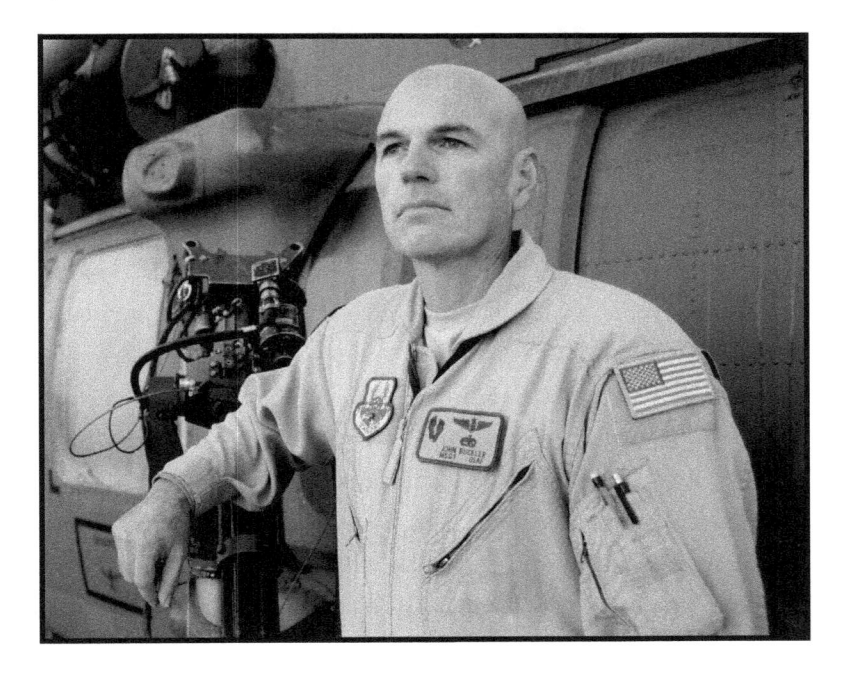

During his career as a Flight Engineer in Combat Search and Rescue he was credited with saving the lives of five wounded servicemen. In addition to receiving several "firewall five" ratings (the highest you can get) during his 26 years in the Air Force, he earned three

Associate's degrees in Applied Sciences; Avionics Technology, Aviation Operations and Professional Aeronautics, a Bachelor's of Science Degree along with an Airframe and Power Plant license and Federal Communications license.

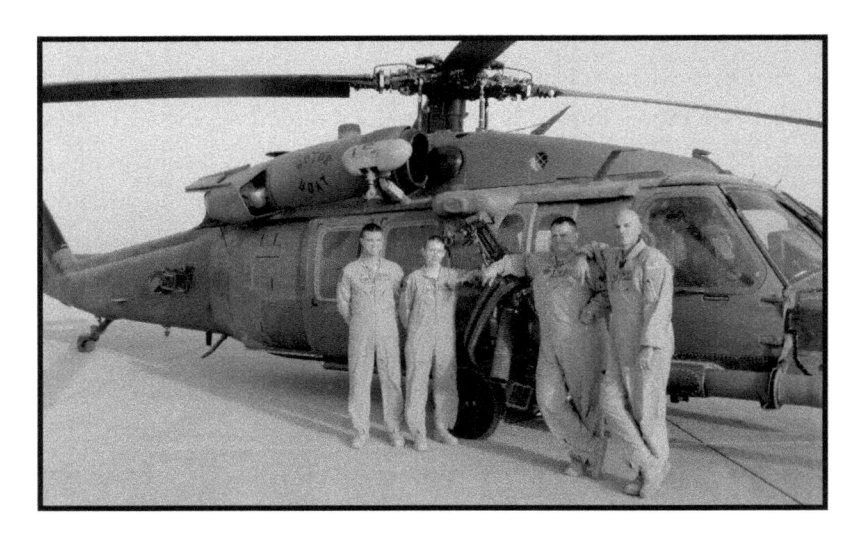

John has been awarded the Air Medal w/three oak leaf clusters - Aerial Achievement Medal w/one oak leaf cluster - Commendation Medal w/two oak leaf clusters - Achievement Medal w/two oak leaf clusters - Combat Readiness Medal w/one oak leaf cluster - Good Conduct Medal w/seven oak leaf clusters - National Defense Service Medal w/one bronze star - Expeditionary Medal - Service Medal w/two bronze stars - Afghanistan Campaign Medal w/one bronze star - Iraq Campaign Medal with one bronze star - Global War on Terrorism Expeditionary Medal - Global War on Terrorism Service Medal - Kuwait Liberation Medal of Kingdom of Saudi Arabia - Kuwait Liberation Medal Government of Kuwait. He also received several letters from his Commanding Officers highly recommending his retention when he was fighting to stay in the Air Force while enduring cancer treatments.

To say John enjoyed what he did in the Air Force is an understatement. He loved it and was very good at it.

Seven years later, after having been told his career was more than likely over, he retired from the United States Air Force.

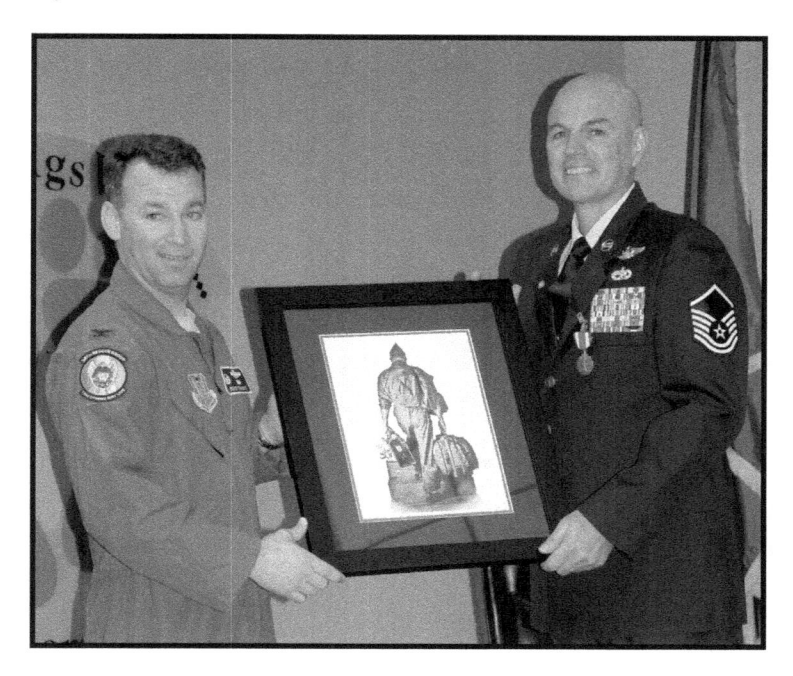

After he retired John decided he wanted to go to school to learn the fine art of cabinet and furniture making. He found a great school in the North Bennet Street School in Boston. He spent two years there and graduated with a degree in his field. He made several pieces while there plus made some pieces he was able to sell.

One of his goals is to travel to the national parks in the US. He has made it to a couple so far but something always comes up which prevents him from starting the big trip. His travel trailer was in pretty bad shape so he bought a different one. This time a fifth wheel. Not a new one but a different one. Now that one is in need of some repairs before he can start on his next adventure.

Then the truck he had in San Antonio was beginning to drain him financially, so he sold that one and bought a brand new one. With John, there is always something.

John still suffers from significant hearing loss. He has hearing aids but even with those he, at times, has difficulty comprehending what is being said. He also still has a difficult time swallowing. He drinks lots of liquids while eating to make it easier for him to swallow. And his mouth is very sensitive to spice. There is very little spice he can tolerate. Having said all this, he is alive and healthy with no more signs of the cancer that afflicted him in 2005. For that, we are forever indebted to the care he was given at Wilford Hall by the United States Air Force and to the grace of God.

Just recently John was honored as a Hometown Hero by the Cincinnati Red's Baseball organization during the game and on his 60th birthday.

John currently lives in Georgia but manages to come north to visit often.

CATHERINE BUCKLER

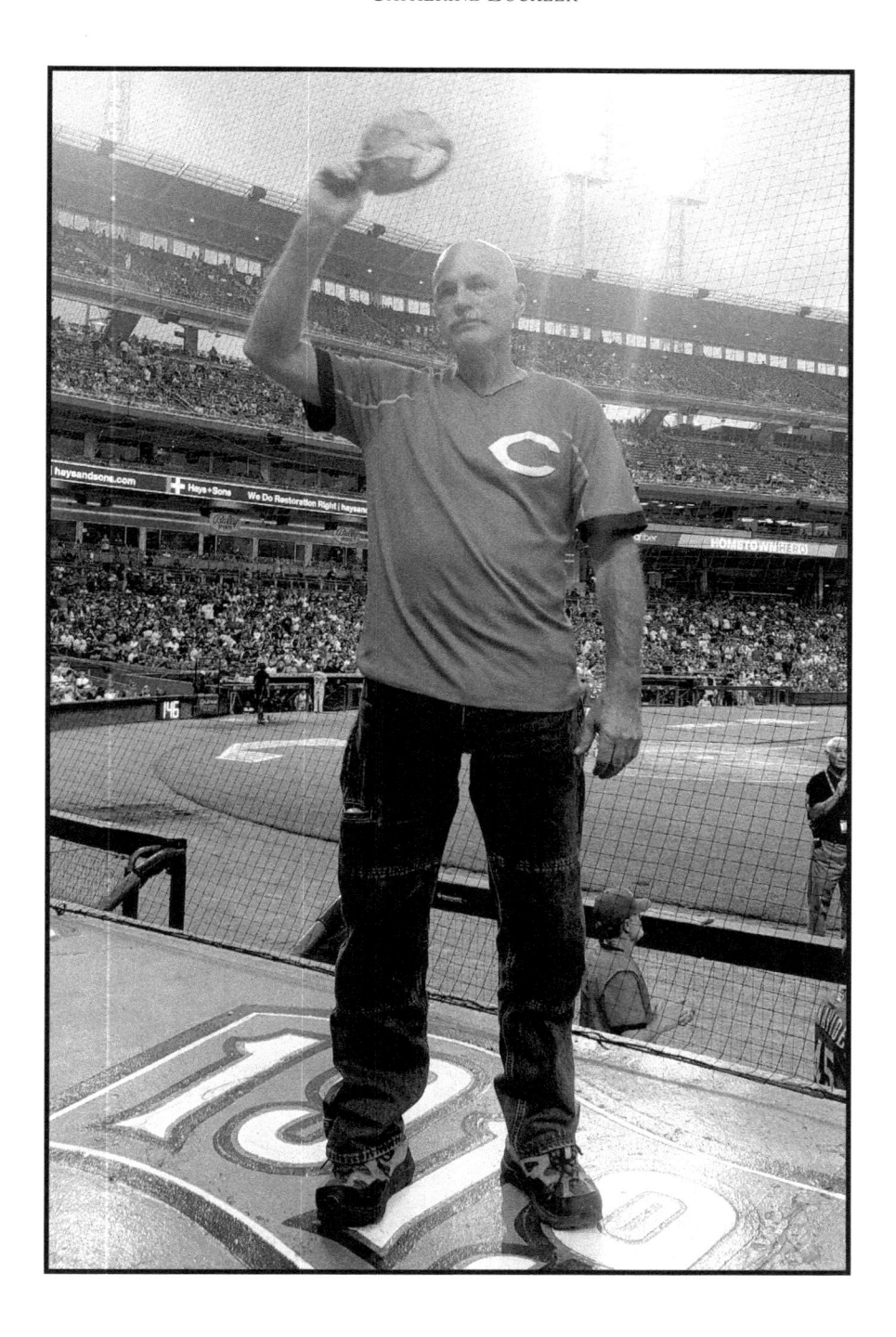

ACKNOWLEDGMENTS

First and foremost, I must acknowledge John who went through an incredible amount of pain, discomfort, challenges, super highs and significant lows. When I would get frustrated by the bureaucracy, he usually responded, "Mom, I have been going through this for nearly 20 years. Get used to it!" As you have read, he never once really complained. He might have moaned groaned, winced, gotten teary but never, ever complained or asked "Why me?" He truly lives, even today, by his squadron's motto: "These Things We Do, That Others May Live."

My friends from 2005 and those more recently, who stated "I cannot leave work on Friday until I get your emails." "You should write a book about John's experiences." first planted the seed of putting the emails into book form.

My dear, dear friend Winkie Foster without whose tenacity, persistence, encouragement, suggestions, support and editing, this book would never have been written. I will be forever grateful.

Ann Schlinkert, who recently asked questions about John and when he retired. I answered "Seven years later." Ann's response was "That's the title of your book!" That statement motivated me to complete the work which had been lingering for more than ten years.

Our daughters, Roxanne, Tracy and Marjorie who read, re-read, made suggestions, critiqued, encouraged, and through the years during other "events" had my back any time I needed them. They may never know how much their support meant to me.

My husband, Ray who's never ending, "if that's what you want to do, it's ok with me!" allows me free reign during our lifetime together. He also never complains about anything and has always has been my biggest supporter.

Printed in the USA
CPSIA information can be obtained
at www.ICGtesting.com
LVHW011648090324
773807LV00013B/401